Acute Exacerbation
of
Respiratory Diseases

CLINICAL FOCUS SERIES

Acute Exacerbation
of
Respiratory Diseases

Steven A Sahn MD

Professor of Medicine and Director
Division of Pulmonary,
Critical Care, Allergy and Sleep Medicine
Medical University of South Carolina
Charleston, South Carolina, USA

JAYPEE BROTHERS MEDICAL PUBLISHERS (P) LTD.

New Delhi • Panama City • London

Jaypee Brothers Medical Publishers (P) Ltd.

Headquarters

Jaypee Brothers Medical Publishers (P) Ltd.
4838/24, Ansari Road, Daryaganj
New Delhi 110 002, India
Phone: +91-11-43574357
Fax: +91-11-43574314
Email: jaypee@jaypeebrothers.com

JP Medical Ltd.
83, Victoria Street, London
SW1H 0HW (UK)
Phone: +44-2031708910
Fax: +02-03-0086180
Email: info@jpmedpub.com

Jaypee-Highlights Medical Publishers Inc.
City of Knowledge, Bld. 237, Clayton
Panama City, Panama
Phone: +507-317-0160
Fax: +50-73-010499
Email: cservice@jphmedical.com

Website: www.jaypeebrothers.com
Website: www.jaypeedigital.com

© 2012, Jaypee Brothers Medical Publishers

Inquiries for bulk sales may be solicited at: jaypee@jaypeebrothers.com

This book has been published in good faith that the contents provided by the author(s) contained herein are original, and is intended for educational purposes only. While every effort is made to ensure accuracy of information, the publisher and the author(s) specifically disclaim any damage, liability, or loss incurred, directly or indirectly, from the use or application of any of the contents of this work. If not specifically stated, all figures and tables are courtesy of the author(s). Where appropriate, the readers should consult with a specialist or contact the manufacturer of the drug or device.

Publisher: Jitendar P Vij
Publishing Director: Tarun Duneja
Editors: Shaila Prashar, DC Gupta, Neeraj Choudhary, Naren Aggarwal
Cover Design: Sachin Dhawan, Seema Dogra

Clinical Focus Series
Acute Exacerbation of Respiratory Diseases / Steven A Sahn
First Edition: **2012**

ISBN-13: 978-93-5025-267-3

Printed in India Sanat Printers, Kundli.

CONTENTS

Contributing Authors

Sonia Bains MD
Assistant Professor of Medicine
Division of Pulmonary, Critical Care,
Allergy and Sleep Medicine
Medical University of South Carolina
Charleston, South Carolina, USA

Patrick A Flume MD
Professor of Medicine
Director of the Cystic Fibrosis Center
Division of Pulmonary, Critical Care,
Allergy and Sleep Medicine
Medical University of South Carolina
Charleston, South Carolina, USA

J Terril Huggins MD
Assistant Professor of Medicine
Division of Pulmonary, Critical Care,
Allergy and Sleep Medicine
Medical University of South Carolina
Charleston, South Carolina, USA

Marc A Judson MD
Professor of Medicine and Chief
Division of Pulmonary and Critical Care
Medicine, Department of Medicine
Albany Medical College
Albany, New York, USA

Lawrence Mohr MD
Professor of Medicine
Environmental Biosciences Program
and Department of Medicine
Medical University of South Carolina
Charleston, South Carolina, USA

Efstratios Panselinas MD
Pulmonary Department
General Army Hospital
Tripoli, Greece

Vlassis Polychronopoulos MD
Director, Third Chest Department
Sismanoglion Hospital
Athens, Greece

Steven A Sahn MD
Professor of Medicine and Director
Division of Pulmonary, Critical Care,
Allergy and Sleep Medicine
Medical University of South Carolina
Charleston, South Carolina, USA

Charlie Strange MD
Professor of Medicine
Division of Pulmonary, Critical Care,
Allergy and Sleep Medicine
Medical University of South Carolina
Charleston, South Carolina, USA

Timothy PM Whelan MD
Associate Professor of Medicine
Medical Director of Adult Lung
Transplantation Program
Medical University of South Carolina
Charleston, South Carolina, USA

PREFACE

The medical dictionary defines "acute" as referring to a health effect that is brief and not chronic, and sometimes, loosely used to mean severe. In referring to exposure, it may be brief, intense, short-term, or of high intensity. An exacerbation is defined as an increase in the severity of a disease that may have its onset rapidly over one or two hour time-frame as in asthma, over a few days as in COPD, or more insidious over several days or weeks, as in cystic fibrosis and non-cystic fibrosis bronchiectasis. These exacerbations may be more insidious, as in IPF and sarcoidosis. Drug-induced adverse effects can be observed over a spectrum from an acute hypersensitivity reaction, or more commonly, an insidious change in the respiratory status that can vary in intensity and duration of exposure. In IPF, the typical time of the "acute exacerbation" varies from one to four weeks and results in significant mortality. A pulmonary exacerbation of sarcoidosis needs to be differentiated from other respiratory illnesses, as their treatments would be different. Classification of hypersensitivity pneumonitis (HP) into acute, subacute, and chronic forms can be misleading, as the clinical findings often overlap in a particular individual. Acute HP, in a previously undiagnosed individual typically begins relatively soon after exposure within hours with respiratory and constitutional symptoms; while a sub-acute or chronic exacerbation tends to be more insidious. As the number of lung transplants continues to increase, clinicians will have to address the significant number of medical and surgical issues that impact the patient's survival. Today, as compared to 20 years ago, clinicians now have a number of tools to manage diverse problems, such as acute and chronic rejection. Hopefully, in the not too distant future, there will be an ideal immunosuppressive agent that will prevent rejection and not lead to severe, often fatal infection.

As you read through this book, you will become aware of differences and similarities between an onset and severity of acute exacerbations in different diseases. I hope that this information will enable clinicians to recognize and appropriately manage patients with acute exacerbations of a respiratory disease.

Steven A Sahn

Acute Exacerbations of COPD

Charlie Strange

EPIDEMIOLOGY

Chronic obstructive pulmonary disease (COPD) is a common lung disease, which is defined by fixed obstruction on spirometry.[1] Since most of the world does not use spirometry, regularly across the affected population, methods like questionaires, have been used in national health surveys to establish the prevalence of disease. Using questionnaires to ask about the prevalence of chronic bronchitis or emphysema, the National Health Interview Survey found 10 million adults in the United States during 2000 affected with this disease.[2] Underdiagnosis is prominent in every recent survey performed. Therefore, when the Third National Health and Nutrition Examination Survey (NHANES III) performed spirometry, it was possible to extrapolate that 23.6 million individuals have COPD in the United States. Importantly, 2.4 million of these had severe or very severe disease with forced expiratory volume in 1 second (FEV_1) less than 50% of the predicted, representing 1.4% of the population.[3] This severely impaired population is the group which has the majority of diagnosed COPD exacerbations.

COPD is poorly recognized throughout the world. Instead, most of the world recognizes chronic bronchitis more often than COPD.[4] In a 2002 health survey, administered by the World Health Organization, only 15% of Americans and fewer individuals from Germany, China and Brazil were able to identify COPD as a disease of the lungs.[4] The misdiagnosis is not helped by the International Classification of Disease (ICD 9 and ICD 10) descriptions of COPD that code COPD into a variety of overlapping categories. Chronic bronchitis has been characterized as the most common phenotype of COPD throughout the past 30 years. However, when chronic bronchitis is defined as a chronic productive cough for three months from each of two successive years, there is an increased recognition that some individuals will not have concomitant airflow obstruction. Therefore, current understanding is that airflow obstruction is necessary to define the disease accurately.

An acute exacerbation of COPD is a major cause of morbidity, the need for urgent care, hospitalization, and mortality. However, very few patients know the meaning of the word exacerbation. In an international study, Kessler et al. found that

1.6% of individuals with advanced COPD knew the meaning of the term and instead preferred terms such as crisis (16%) or infection (20%).[5] Nevertheless, the definitions and terminology used for an acute exacerbation of COPD have now been sufficiently codified to suggest that a change in terminology is unlikely to occur.

CASE STUDY 1

MS is a 64-year-old woman who presents for a first office visit because of cough and purulent sputum of four days duration. On careful questioning, she noted that she could not go on hikes during summer vacation in the mountains because of the high altitude and older age. She first started smoking at the age of 20 and continued smoking one pack daily. She admits to have a "smoker's cough" on awakening most mornings, but this usually clears after her morning shower. All she wants from today's visit is an antibiotic because her sputum is now yellow and she noted dyspnea throughout the day, yesterday.

On examination, she is afebrile; vital signs are normal. Chest auscultation reveals polyphonic wheezing in all lung fields. The remainder of the examination is normal.

Spirometry in the office shows FEV_1 of 1.5 L (46% predicted), forced vital capacity (FVC) of 2.7 L (72% predicted) and $FEV_1/FVC = 0.56$. A chest radiograph is clear.

What is Her Diagnosis? Should Other Testing Be Done?

MS has an acute exacerbation of COPD. The first presentation of COPD is often precipitated by an exacerbation. Spirometry is essential to establish a diagnosis of COPD. To exclude asthma, spirometry will need to be repeated after optimal care with inhaled bronchodilators and corticosteroid medications. If spirometry returns to normal, the diagnosis of asthma can be established. In individuals over the age of 40 with a significant smoking history, the more likely diagnosis is COPD that will be proven by persistent obstruction on repeated spirometry at a return visit. A common mistake is to miss the opportunity to establish the diagnosis of obstructive airways disease (COPD or asthma) at the first visit when a patient is requesting antibiotics. Spirometry, 20 minutes following administration of albuterol in the office, may show some improvement in either COPD or asthma. Only if spirometry returns to normal ($FEV_1/FVC > 0.7$ and $FEV_1 > 80\%$ predicted), a diagnosis of asthma can be definitively established.

CURRENT DEFINITION

An acute exacerbation of COPD was first established by Anthonison as a clinical worsening of at least two of the following three symptoms: worsened dyspnea, worsened sputum volume, and change in sputum color.[6] Since the majority of the patients met the clinical definition of chronic bronchitis and the Anthonison's study demonstrated some role for antibiotics in treatment, the subsequent literature became adulterated with terminology that used the term "acute exacerbation of chronic bronchitis" (AECB). This term continues to be used by the United States Food and Drug Administration to define antibiotics effective for upper respiratory infections. The association with infection has persisted in most perceptions about the disease. This chapter will suggest that patients with AECB receive spirometry to define and stage COPD, but will hereafter use the terminology acute exacerbation of COPD that has an evidence-based therapy.

The global initiative for chronic obstructive lung disease (GOLD) guidelines currently define an acute exacerbation of COPD as an event in the natural course of the disease characterized by a change in the patient's baseline dyspnea, cough with or without sputum that is beyond normal day-to-day variation, is acute in onset, and may warrant a change in medication in a patient with underlying COPD.[1] As a result, much effort has been expended on measuring the diseased state accurately and accounting for the daily variability in symptoms. Therefore, accurate diagnosis of an exacerbation of COPD requires use of spirometry to first diagnose COPD, since treatment of individuals with bronchitic symptoms without obstruction can lead to overdiagnosis.

CLINICAL ATTRIBUTES OF A COPD EXACERBATION

Recent interest in therapies designed to decrease exacerbations has helped to focus the specifics of the definition. Unfortunately, the anatomy of an exacerbation has significant variability in most domains. In part, this variability is dependent on the severity and the phenotype of COPD. Additionally, exacerbations can be defined on the basis of clinical grounds or healthcare utilization, recognizing that more than 30% of exacerbations are not reported to a healthcare professional.[7]

Individuals with COPD on an average have 1–4 exacerbations yearly; however, the frequency is dependent on past exacerbation frequency and severity of COPD.[8] Exacerbations can be measured by number, time to first exacerbation, duration of exacerbation, or intensity of exacerbation. However, the best measure to study for clinical trials is based on the event frequency and the variability in that event measurement.

Most of the individuals with COPD have day-to-day variability in symptoms that is poorly understood. Individuals with chronic bronchitis have more airway hyperresponsiveness and may be more susceptible to an exacerbation than individuals with emphysema. Nevertheless, the burden of a given exacerbation is likely no different between these subgroups of COPD. Instead, COPD exacerbation symptoms and healthcare utilization are closely related to baseline health status.

Unfortunately, uniform definitions of an acute exacerbation of COPD have not been prospectively validated. Although symptom-based definitions are popular, it has been recognized that patients under-report exacerbation frequency by approximately 50%.[9] Newer attempts to prospectively validate whether symptoms are worse than day-to-day variation have been proposed. The most recent new instruments to define the frequency and severity of COPD exacerbations have been the exacerbations of chronic pulmonary disease tool (EXACT) questionnaire[10] and the COPD assessment tool (CAT).[11] These new tools are currently in the validation stages.

HEALTHCARE UTILIZATION

COPD exacerbations are responsible for physician visits, emergency room visits, hospitalizations, intensive care unit (ICU) admissions, respiratory failure and mechanical ventilation days, and death.

Indirect costs include days unable to perform usual activities and premature disability. In one study, disability between ages of 40 years and 63 years occurred in 22.8% of diagnosed COPD patients as compared to 7.3% of the remainder of the population.[12]

The sum of these costs varies throughout the world. Annual societal costs in 2002 ranged from US$ 1,361 in the Netherlands to US$ 6,475 in Spain.[13] Additionally, the costs associated with the last 6 months of life appear higher for COPD than for lung cancer.[14] The majority of these costs are with COPD exacerbation treatment.

PATHOPHYSIOLOGY

The inflamed airway of COPD is of multifactorial etiology. Polymorphonuclear (PMN) predominant airways cellularity is induced by cigarette smoking; however, this PMN predominant inflammation persists despite smoking cessation. Mucous gland hypertrophy leading to mucous hypersecretion, airway wall thickening, and transition of the airway to have persistent bacterial colonization, are all part of COPD pathogenesis.

The etiology of a COPD exacerbation remains incompletely understood. However, most evidence suggests that acute airways inflammation occurs on top of the chronic neutrophilic airways inflammation. PMN and eosinophils have been found in bronchial tissue.[15,16] Elevations of IL-6, fibrinogen, C-reactive protein, and procalcitonin have been found in airways and serum, suggesting systemic inflammation.[17,18] In short, most of the efforts have been spent on characterizing the cause of inflammation, recognizing that the two most likely etiologies are microbial and environmental for which there is limited therapy.

Bacterial exacerbations of COPD have traditionally been characterized when sputum purulence is prominent. *Haemophilus influenzae, Moraxella catarrhalis* and *Streptococcus pneumoniae* appear to be the predominant initiating pathogens.[19]

However, many different serotypes of each pathogen can incite specific adaptive immune responses that typically peak at 4–8 weeks after the acquisition of a new bacterial strain. Additionally, some strains of acquired bacteria adhere to airway epithelial cells and elicit IL-8 in higher levels than other strains.[20] The immune response, which elicits antibodies that bind to the bacterial cell surface, is also highly strain specific.[21] Therefore, recurrent exacerbations can occur with small differences in surface antigen presentation with the same bacterial species.

The consequences of airways inflammation are worsened mucosal edema, airway secretions, and bronchospasm. Then ventilation-perfusion mismatch and dyspnea occur followed by cough, dyspnea, sputum production, and these lead to worsened quality of life. Patient perception, access to care, and physician's interpretation of symptoms then become the variables that define subsequent course.

In addition to bacterial infection, environmental factors play a role in some exacerbations. Airway injuries from chemical inhalation, industrial pollutants, and allergens have been identified as causes for some acute exacerbations of COPD. A history of exposure, eosinophilic airways inflammation, and less systemic inflammatory symptoms suggest these causes.[1] The hunt for environmental causes of exacerbations is occasionally worthwhile, particularly when IgE-mediated allergens are involved. Thus, study of the impact of oral and inhaled corticosteroid therapy on COPD exacerbations is complicated by the need to systematically account for overlap populations with allergic disease.

Viral infections also play a role in acute exacerbations of COPD. Many prospective studies have been performed that used highly sensitive techniques of polymerase chain reaction (PCR) with or without reverse transcriptase PCR to define viral presence during exacerbations. A recent meta-analysis[22] has suggested that 34.1% (95% CI: 23.9–44.4) of acute exacerbations were associated with viral pathogens. The specific viruses implicated included picornavirus 17.3% (95% CI: 7.2–27.3), influenza 7.4% (95% CI: 2.9–12.0), respiratory syncytial virus 5.3% (95% CI: 1.6–9.0), corona viruses 3.1% (95% CI: 0.4–5.8), parainfluenza 2.6% (95% CI: 0.4–4.8), adenovirus 1.1% (95% CI: –1.1–3.3), and human metapneumovirus 0.7% (95% CI: –0.3–1.8). Unfortunately, the systemic response to viral infections is similar to bacterial infections. Biomarker development to discriminate the cause of acute exacerbations has not been optimized. Serum procalcitonin and C-reactive protein (CRP) are not different between viral and nonviral causes of exacerbations.[23]

Influenza vaccination with the trivalent split virion vaccine has been demonstrated in some studies to lower the healthcare utilization for severe COPD patients through less hospital presentations, episodes of pneumonia, and intensive care unit stays.[24] Although the immunological response to vaccination may not be as robust in a COPD population as in others without systemic illness, the benefits are sufficient to make influenza vaccination a standard of care for all COPD patients.

CASE STUDY 2

JP is a 70-year-old patient with GOLD stage IV COPD with FEV_1 = 28% predicted. Over the past year, he has experienced four exacerbations requiring office visits. On these occasions, he was treated with a seven-day-course of oral prednisone, an increase in his prescribed albuterol dose and an oral antibiotic for 10 days. Doxycycline, amoxicillin-clavulanate, and trimethoprim-sulfamethoxazole, all have been used with success. He states compliance with tiotropium, beta-2 agonists, and inhaled corticosteroid therapy.

Yesterday, he noted the onset of fever after having five days of clinical worsening. He was thinking about coming to the office on Friday, but decided to wait until Monday to show up because of the weekend. He describes his mucus as thick green and more copious in volume over the last week. Yesterday, he estimated that half cup of mucus has been expectorated in 24 hours.

On examination, his temperature is 38 °C and vital signs are otherwise normal. He can speak in full sentences and has no accessory muscle use. Lung examination reveals wheezing, prolonged expiratory phase, and no consolidation. A chest radiograph is normal, excepting a mild increase in interstitial markings at both lung bases.

What is His Diagnosis? Should Sputum Cultures Be Performed? Would a Chest CT Scan Change Management?

JP has another acute exacerbation of COPD despite stated compliance with the best medications available to prevent COPD exacerbations. There are few studies that address the optimal care of the patient with frequent exacerbations; however, most pulmonary specialists take such opportunities and further explore additional possible causes.

The differential diagnosis of the patient with frequent exacerbations includes environmental, anatomical, and microbial causes. A careful examination of hobbies and recreational activities should focus on fumes or particulate exposures. Concomitant asthma and allergic rhinitis can coexist. Therefore, serum-IgE measurement with or without a search for aeroallergens, including pets, dust mites, and cockroach allergy, are reasonable.

Sputum culture in JP subsequently showed *Pseudomonas aeruginosa*. *Pseudomonas* colonization has been found in significant numbers of GOLD IV COPD subjects. When present, *Pseudomonas* colonization is associated with more frequent exacerbations. Efficacy of oral therapy is variable and depends on sensitivities that should be performed if *Pseudomonas* is isolated.

Pseudomonas colonization is seen more frequently in the COPD patient with bronchiectasis. Both frequent exacerbations with or without the culture of a Gram-negative enteric organism are reasons to obtain a noncontrast chest computed tomography (CT) scan. Bronchiectasis has been found on CT of COPD patients in up to 40 percent of cases. Depending on the focality and distribution, additional studies are warranted if not previously performed. Acquired quantitative deficiencies of immunoglobulins can be seen in COPD populations. Allergic bronchopulmonary aspergillosis (ABPA) can be diagnosed and treated. Alfa-1 antitrypsin deficiency can also have severe bronchiectasis, in part secondary to concomitant colonization with *Mycobacterium avium* complex.

Therefore, the management of JP is changed by obtaining sputum cultures and a chest CT scan.

CLINICAL IMPACT

Symptoms

Cough, sputum production, and dyspnea are the core symptoms of a COPD acute exacerbation. Cough frequency, cough severity, and sputum volume remain quite difficult outcomes to systematically capture. Dyspnea has well-validated tools for clinical assessment for both baseline and transitional dyspnea indices; however, dyspnea occurs more commonly in patients with advanced COPD and does not occur in milder disease. Recently, the breathlessness, cough, and sputum severity (BCSS) instrument has been used to measure chronic COPD symptoms.[25] This instrument is not designed to measure the severity or define the frequency of acute exacerbations.

Emergency Room Care and Hospitalization

Both emergency room (ER) utilization and hospitalization for acute exacerbation are significant events in the life of a COPD patient. Exacerbation rates are not linear over time in all patients with COPD. The first ER visit or hospitalization increases the risk of a second event and is a marker of significant one year mortality. The number and frequency of exacerbations have been the subjects of many studies since those outcomes correlate to mortality and quality of life.

The annual rate of COPD exacerbations, requiring ER or hospital care, is related to the GOLD stage of COPD. Recently, the addition of other clinical parameters in addition to FEV_1 has allowed better estimates of exacerbation risk. In a recent study of the BODE score, Marin et al.[26] showed that the annual rate of COPD exacerbations was 1.95 (95% CI: 0.90–2.1) in this COPD population. However, the mean time to a first exacerbation was inversely proportional to the worsening of the BODE quartiles (7.9 years, 5.7 years, 3.4 years, and 1.3 years for BODE scores of 0–2, 3–4, 5–6, and 7–10, respectively). Similarly, the mean time to a first COPD emergency room visit was 6.7 years, 3.6 years, 2.0 years, and 0.8 years for BODE quartiles.

Hospital outcomes of patients admitted for an acute exacerbation of COPD are also heterogeneous. In one recent series of 282 patients, 28 patients (9.9%) died during hospitalization, 241 patients (85.5%) were discharged to home, and 13 patients (4.6%) needed long-term care. Survival for two years was over 50%, although quality of life was poor.[27] Living alone may be an independent predictor of hospitalization.

Quality of Life

Quality of life in COPD has most often been measured by the disease-specific St George's respiratory questionnaire (SGRQ). The SGRQ was devised for patients with stable chronic bronchitis and was designed with a recall period of 1–12 months. Other disease specific questionnaires include the chronic respiratory disease questionnaire (CRQ), and the baseline and transitional dyspnea index (BDI, TDI). CRQ and the SGRQ appear to be acceptable to patients during acute exacerbation. However, the recall period of the SGRQ symptom component should be shortened if used during acute exacerbation.[28]

Quality of life is often poor after a COPD exacerbation. The study to understand prognoses and preferences for outcomes and risk of treatments (SUPPORT) prospectively evaluated 1,016 individuals with COPD admitted to the hospital with a $pCO_2 > 50$ mmHg. At six months, only 26% of the cohort were able to rate a good, very good, or excellent quality of life.[29]

Mortality

The mortality following a COPD exacerbation requiring hospitalization is unexpectedly high. Risk factors for high mortality include age, severity of COPD, extent of comorbidities, and intensive care unit admission. In one large study, the one year mortality of COPD exacerbations admitted to the ICU in individuals over the age of 65 years was 59%.[30] Most studies have shown that need for mechanical ventilation is not a strong predictor of subsequent survival, although repeated need for mechanical ventilation is a more ominous event. Although exacerbations of COPD currently rank as the fourth most common cause of death in the United States, few studies have been performed with all cause mortality as the endpoint.

TREATMENT

Outcomes of acute exacerbations are related to the treatment received. Early treatment is associated with faster recovery time. Failure to report an exacerbation to a physician is associated with more hospitalization. Quality of life also appears better when exacerbations are treated as compared to a population with more untreated events.[7] A number of large studies have been performed and analyzed in an attempt to both prevent exacerbations from occurring and optimize treatment of the exacerbation. Statements from the 2009 GOLD guidelines concerning COPD exacerbations are given in table 1-1.[1]

Table 1-1	GOLD Guideline Statements Concerning COPD Exacerbation[1]	
Recommendation	Specific statement	Grade
Monitoring	Frequency, severity, likely causes of exacerbations, and psychological wellbeing should be monitored.	*
Prevention	An inhaled glucocorticosteroid combined with an inhaled beta-2 agonist is more effective than the individual components in reducing exacerbations.	A
Treatment	Inhaled bronchodilators (particularly inhaled beta-2 agonists with or without anticholinergics) and oral gluco-corticosteroids are effective treatments for exacerbations of COPD.	A
Antibiotics	Patients experiencing COPD exacerbations with clinical signs of airway infection (e.g., increased sputum purulence) may benefit from antibiotic treatment.	B
Ventilation	Noninvasive mechanical ventilation in exacerbations improves respiratory acidosis, increases pH, decreases the need for endotracheal intubation, and reduces $PaCO_2$, respiratory rate, severity of breathlessness, the length of hospital stay, and mortality.	A

*Not graded.

Bronchodilators

In COPD exacerbations, bronchodilators improve lung function, reduce symptoms, and when administered chronically, decrease the rate of subsequent exacerbations. These benefits appear to be present with both beta-agonist and anticholinergic bronchodilators, and occur when bronchodilators are administered on top of inhaled corticosteroid therapy.[31] A large study of adding salmeterol to tiotropium found no additional benefit in the reduction of exacerbation frequency, although lung function was marginally better and fewer hospitalizations were recorded compared to tiotropium alone.[32] Few studies have been performed on the optimal dose or dosing frequency of bronchodilators during COPD exacerbations with robust study endpoints. COPD exacerbation outcome is not different between albuterol 2.5 mg and 5.0 mg by nebulizer every 4 hours.[33] However, nebulized bronchodilators using significantly higher doses than bronchodilators administered by metered dose inhalers have been shown to have a marginal benefit during periods of clinical worsening.[34]

Corticosteroids

A few randomized controlled trials of oral or parenteral corticosteroids for COPD exacerbations, which adequately control for other variables, have been performed.

A 2001 Cochrane review of seven such studies suggested that lung function was improved for 72 hours after the initiation of corticosteroids[35] with some studies suggesting that the rate of treatment failure is less. A Veterans Administration cooperative study randomized a hospitalized COPD exacerbation cohort to placebo, short-term corticosteroids (2 weeks), or long-term corticosteroids (8 weeks). The rate of treatment failure was worse for the placebo arm and not different for the two corticosteroid arms.[36]

The dose and mode of corticosteroid delivery remains controversial. Recognizing that oral corticosteroids are 95% bioavailable within a short timeframe, oral dosing of corticosteroids for COPD exacerbations has achieved some favor. Recent propensity adjusted database studies suggest no difference in outcome between orally administered and intravenously administered corticosteroid dosing;[37] however, more studies are clearly needed.

Studies using inhaled corticosteroids have also been performed. Inhaled corticosteroids reduce the rate of exacerbations compared to placebo, predominantly in patients with FEV_1 percent predicted values < 50%.[38] Combination of corticosteroid and beta-agonist inhalers shows reduced frequency of moderate and severe exacerbations than long-acting beta agonist inhalers alone[39,40] or inhaled corticosteroids alone.[40] However, corticosteroid treatment of an existing exacerbation should usually be treated with oral or parenteral corticosteroids since the dose-response curve of inhaled corticosteroids is relatively flat.

Antibiotics

Antibiotics improve the time until COPD exacerbation recovery in most antibiotic studies performed. A recent study has shown that the addition of doxycycline to systemic corticosteroids improved the rate of clinical cure by day 10. Microbiological clearance and symptom scores were better; use of open label antibiotics was less. However, like most of the studies, eventual recovery of the patient at 30 days was not different.[41]

With data suggesting that new strains of bacterial organisms are associated with COPD exacerbations, there is interest in defining if antibiotics and microbial cure suppress subsequent acute exacerbations. One recent large study with 842 patients found a longer time between exacerbations when antibiotics were used for the index exacerbation with the beneficial effects seen mostly in the first 3 months following treatment (hazard ratio 0.72, 95% confidence interval 0.62–0.83). In addition, adding antibiotics to oral corticosteroids reduced the risk of all-cause mortality.[42]

Antibiotics should be targeted to the new bacterial species responsible for the exacerbation, if known. Unfortunately, respiratory tract cultures are difficult to perform since many of the bacterial organisms can also colonize the mouth. Antibiotic use is also complicated by the frequency of *Pseudomonas* species in the flora of some advanced COPD patients.[43]

Mucolytics and Expectorants

Mucolytics and expectorants have been used for many years to treat symptoms of excess mucus. Guaifenesin has been labeled as possibly effective by the US Food and Drug Administration; however, few trials have been done to define if therapy improves any aspect of a COPD exacerbation. Mucus viscosity is less, but possibly at the cost of excess production of mucus. Therefore, guaifenesin preparations have most commonly been used for short-term.

N-acetylcysteine (NAC) has been studied more robustly because of its efficacy as an antioxidant. Most studies have been done with oral formulations used to prevent exacerbations. A recent meta-analysis that incorporated more than 2,000 patients reported that NAC reduced the odds of COPD patients experiencing one or more exacerbations over the treatment period [odds ratio = 0.49, 95% confidence interval (0.32–0.74), p = 0.001]. Treatment effect was preserved in the presence of active smoking and lessened when used with concomitant inhaled corticosteroids.[44] In fact, mucolytics are quite commonly prescribed during a COPD exacerbation in some parts of the world.[45]

Noninvasive Ventilation

A comprehensive discussion of noninvasive ventilation as a treatment strategy for COPD exacerbations is beyond the scope of this chapter. However, this is one of the category A recommendations of the GOLD guidelines at the time of hospitalization when significant hypercapnia is present. Home outpatient use of bilevel positive airway pressure (BIPAP) remains more controversial and is reserved for severely compromized COPD patients.

Self-management

Self-management involves a systematic approach to disease-specific education for COPD patients. Typical programs are focused on early treatment of exacerbations and often are added to exercise-based pulmonary rehabilitation. A recent review of this literature suggests that self-management reduces hospital admissions and marginally improves quality of life; primarily through the reduction in dyspnea.[46] Further work is required to refine self-management programs so that optimal information can be standardized to get these health improvements.

CASE STUDY 3

MT is a 61-year-old female with advanced GOLD IV COPD with FEV_1 = 22% predicted. She presents with worsened dyspnea, unresponsive to three days of oral prednisone at 40 mg daily. She has a worsened cough, but is making no mucus. She denies fever, but her family notes intermittent confusion.

On examination, she is oriented to person and place. Temperature is 37 °C, pulse rate is 110/minute and regular, blood pressure is 136/74, and respiratory rate is 28/minute with accessory muscle use and a prolonged expiratory phase. No wheezing is heard. Breath sounds are distant.

Laboratory examination shows an arterial blood gas with pH 7.18/pCO_2 = 78/ pO_2 = 68 on 4 L nasal O_2 that has been titrated by her home oximeter. A chest radiograph is clear but shows hyperinflation. This was followed by a contrast chest CT that did not show pulmonary embolism. She has not previously been ventilated and desires to do everything possible to keep open her prospects for an upcoming bronchoscopic lung volume reduction procedure.

Initial emergency room therapy included 125 mg intravenous SoluMedrol (methyl prednisolone), nebulized albuterol 5.0 mg, and intravenous broad spectrum antibiotics with cefepime. After 1 hour of emergency room treatment, she is not improved. A repeat ABG shows pH 7.14/pCO_2 = 82/and pO_2 = 64.

Should MT Receive Endotracheal Intubation and Mechanical Ventilation?

Ethically, MT should receive optimal aggressive care for her COPD exacerbation. Although she has advanced COPD, this is her first exacerbation, and the likelihood of dying during this admission is < 20%. In addition, she is a likely candidate for other therapies for COPD including lung transplantation, surgical lung volume reduction, or one of the newer emerging therapies for bronchoscopic volume reduction.

The decision for endotracheal intubation depends on the likelihood that noninvasive mechanical ventilation will reverse the clinical course. Since MT is only 1 hour into aggressive therapy for her COPD, most clinicians would first attempt a trial of mask ventilation using a full facemask. This intervention requires the application of an expiratory positive airway pressure (EPAP) usually beginning with 5–10 cmH_2O pressure that is designed to splint open small airways in collapse. Then inspiratory positive airway pressure is added slowly and titrated to patient comfort. The difference between IPAP and EPAP is the pressure available to assist with ventilation. Standard of care requires measurement of tidal volume and repeated ABG to determine the treatment efficacy since further clinical worsening should prompt endotracheal intubation and mechanical ventilation. Regardless of ventilator strategy, MT should receive care in the intensive care unit.

FUTURE RESEARCH

More precise definition of a COPD exacerbation is one of the goals of the COPD community. Early in this decade it became clear that a paper-based diary was insufficient to adequately characterize exacerbation frequency or severity.[47] Therefore, a large effort is being expended to use electronic capture of home events since early treatment of exacerbations has been shown to improve outcome of COPD exacerbations. The EXACT questionnaire is being distributed by a consortium of software vendors to allow home electronic data capture in a very short period of time, daily. Electronic capture has an advantage over diary cards since each entry is timed. When coupled with medication delivery timing devices, a better understanding of the anatomy of a COPD exacerbation will be possible.

Other areas of active research include efforts to better understand the anatomy of large and small airways on CT, oscillometry and optical coherence tomography (OCT).[48] A large effort is attempting to better understand the biological events that lead to persistence of neutrophilic inflammation in the airway after the removal of airway injury such as tobacco smoke. Given the enormity of healthcare utilization for COPD exacerbations, much more research effort and more biologic treatment options are needed to understand this frequent clinical condition.

REFERENCES

1. World Health Organization. Global strategy for diagnosis, management, and prevention of COPD. Available at http://www.goldcopd.com/Guidelineitem asp?l1=2&l2=1&intId=2180 (accessed 6-20-2010) 2009.
2. Mannino DM, Braman S. The epidemiology and economics of chronic obstructive pulmonary disease. *Proc Am Thorac Soc.* 2007;4:502-6.
3. American Lung Association. Chronic Obstructive Pulmonary Disease (COPD) Fact Sheet. Available at http://www.lungusa.org/lung-disease/copd/resources/facts-figures/COPD-Fact-Sheet.html 2010.
4. Rennard S, Decramer M, Calverley PM, et al. Impact of COPD in North America and Europe in 2000: subjects' perspective of Confronting COPD International Survey. *Eur Respir J.* 2002;20:799-805.
5. Kessler R, Stahl E, Vogelmeier C, et al. Patient understanding, detection, and experience of COPD exacerbations: an observational, interview-based study. *Chest.* 2006;130:133-42.
6. Anthonisen NR, Manfreda J, Warren CP, et al. Antibiotic therapy in exacerbations of chronic obstructive pulmonary disease. *Ann Intern Med.* 1987;106:196-204.
7. Wilkinson TM, Donaldson GC, Hurst JR, et al. Early therapy improves outcomes of exacerbations of chronic obstructive pulmonary disease. *Am J Respir Crit Care Med.* 2004;169:1298-303.
8. Anzueto A, Sethi S, Martinez FJ. Exacerbations of chronic obstructive pulmonary disease. *Proc Am Thorac Soc.* 2007;4:554-64.
9. Seemungal TA, Donaldson GC, Bhowmik A, et al. Time course and recovery of exacerbations in patients with chronic obstructive pulmonary disease. *Am J Respir Crit Care Med.* 2000;161:1608-13.

10. Jones P, Higenbottam T. Quantifying of severity of exacerbations in chronic obstructive pulmonary disease: adaptations to the definition to allow quantification. *Proc Am Thorac Soc.* 2007;4:597-601.

11. Jones PW, Harding G, Berry P, et al. Development and first validation of the COPD assessment test. *Eur Respir J.* 2009;34:648-54.

12. Darkow T, Kadlubek PJ, Shah H, et al. A retrospective analysis of disability and its related costs among employees with chronic obstructive pulmonary disease. *J Occup Environ Med.* 2007;49:22-30.

13. Wouters EF. Economic analysis of the Confronting COPD survey: an overview of results. *Respir Med.* 2003;97:S3-14.

14. Au DH, Udris EM, Fihn SD, et al. Differences in health care utilization at the end of life among patients with chronic obstructive pulmonary disease and patients with lung cancer. *Arch Intern Med.* 2006;166:326-31.

15. Zhu J, Qiu YS, Majumdar S, et al. Exacerbations of bronchitis: bronchial eosinophilia and gene expression for interleukin-4, interleukin-5, and eosinophil chemoattractants. *Am J Respir Crit Care Med.* 2001;164:109-16.

16. Papi A, Bellettato CM, Braccioni F, et al. Infections and airway inflammation in chronic obstructive pulmonary disease severe exacerbations. *Am J Respir Crit Care Med.* 2006; 173:1114-21.

17. Wedzicha JA, Donaldson GC. Exacerbations of chronic obstructive pulmonary disease. *Respir Care.* 2003;48:1204-13.

18. Wedzicha JA, Seemungal TA, MacCallum PK, et al. Acute exacerbations of chronic obstructive pulmonary disease are accompanied by elevations of plasma fibrinogen and serum IL-6 levels. *Thromb Haemost.* 2000;84:210-5.

19. Sethi S, Evans N, Grant BJ, et al. New strains of bacteria and exacerbations of chronic obstructive pulmonary disease. *N Engl J Med.* 2002;347:465-71.

20. Chin CL, Manzel LJ, Lehman EE, et al. *Haemophilus influenzae* from patients with chronic obstructive pulmonary disease exacerbation induce more inflammation than colonizers. *Am J Respir Crit Care Med.* 2005;172:85-91.

21. Bogaert D, Van der Valk P, Ramdin R, et al. Host-pathogen interaction during pneumococcal infection in patients with chronic obstructive pulmonary disease. *Infect Immun.* 2004;72:818-23.

22. Mohan A, Chandra S, Agarwal D, et al. Prevalence of viral infection detected by PCR and RT-PCR in patients with acute exacerbation of COPD: a systematic review. *Respirology.* 2010;15:536-42.

23. Kherad O, Kaiser L, Bridevaux PO, et al. Upper respiratory viral infections, biomarkers and chronic obstructive pulmonary disease (COPD) exacerbations. *Chest.* 2010;138:896-904.

24. Anar C, Bicmen C, Yapicioglu S, et al. Evaluation of clinical data and antibody response following influenza vaccination in patients with chronic obstructive pulmonary disease. *New Microbiol.* 2010;33:117-27.

25. Leidy NK, Rennard SI, Schmier J, et al. The breathlessness, cough, and sputum scale: the development of empirically based guidelines for interpretation. *Chest.* 2003;124:2182-91.

26. Marin JM, Carrizo SJ, Casanova C, et al. Prediction of risk of COPD exacerbations by the BODE index. *Respir Med.* 2009;103:373-8.

27. Wang Q, Bourbeau J. Outcomes and health-related quality of life following hospitalization for an acute exacerbation of COPD. *Respirology.* 2005;10:334-40.

28. Doll H, Duprat-Lomon I, Ammerman E, et al. Validity of the St George's respiratory questionnaire at acute exacerbation of chronic bronchitis: comparison with the Nottingham health profile. *Qual Life Res.* 2003;12:117-32.

29. Connors AF, Dawson NV, Thomas C, et al. Outcomes following acute exacerbation of severe chronic obstructive lung disease. The SUPPORT investigators (Study to Understand Prognoses and Preferences for Outcomes and Risks of Treatments). *Am J Respir Crit Care Med.* 1996;154:959-67.

30. Seneff MG, Wagner DP, Wagner RP, et al. Hospital and 1-year survival of patients admitted to intensive care units with acute exacerbation of chronic obstructive pulmonary disease. *JAMA.* 1995;274:1852-7.

31. Suh DC, Lau H, La HO, et al. Association between incidence of acute exacerbation and medication therapy in patients with COPD. *Curr Med Res Opin.* 2010;26:297-306.

32. Aaron SD, Vandemheen KL, Fergusson D, et al. Tiotropium in combination with placebo, salmeterol, or fluticasone-salmeterol for treatment of chronic obstructive pulmonary disease: a randomized trial. *Ann Intern Med.* 2007;146:545-55.

33. Nair S, Thomas E, Pearson SB, et al. A randomized controlled trial to assess the optimal dose and effect of nebulized albuterol in acute exacerbations of COPD. *Chest.* 2005; 128:48-54.

34. O'Driscoll BR, Kay EA, Taylor RJ, et al. A long-term prospective assessment of home nebulizer treatment. *Respir Med.* 1992;86:317-25.

35. Wood-Baker R, Walters EH, Gibson P. Oral corticosteroids for acute exacerbations of chronic obstructive pulmonary disease. *Cochrane Database Syst Rev.* 2001;(2): CD001288. Update in *Cochrane Database Syst Rev.* 2005;(1):CD001288.

36. Erbland ML, Deupree RH, Niewoehner DE. Systemic corticosteroids in chronic obstructive pulmonary disease exacerbations (SCCOPE): rationale and design of an equivalence trial. Veterans Administration Cooperative Trials SCCOPE Study Group. *Control Clin Trials.* 1998;19:404-17.

37. Lindenauer PK, Pekow PS, Lahti MC, et al. Association of corticosteroid dose and route of administration with risk of treatment failure in acute exacerbation of chronic obstructive pulmonary disease. *JAMA.* 2010;303:2359-67.

38. Jones PW, Willits LR, Burge PS, et al. Disease severity and the effect of fluticasone propionate on chronic obstructive pulmonary disease exacerbations. *Eur Respir J.* 2003; 21:68-73.

39. Ferguson GT, Anzueto A, Fei R, et al. Effect of fluticasone propionate/salmeterol (250/50 microg) or salmeterol (50 microg) on COPD exacerbations. *Respir Med.* 2008; 102:1099-108.

40. Calverley PM, Boonsawat W, Cseke Z, et al. Maintenance therapy with budesonide and formoterol in chronic obstructive pulmonary disease. *Eur Respir J.* 2003;22:912-9.

41. Daniels JM, Snijders D, de Graaff CS, et al. Antibiotics in addition to systemic corticosteroids for acute exacerbations of chronic obstructive pulmonary disease. *Am J Respir Crit Care Med.* 2010;181:150-7.

42. Roede BM, Bresser P, Prins JM, et al. Reduced risk of next exacerbation and mortality associated with antibiotic use in COPD. *Eur Respir J.* 2009;33:282-8.

43. Martinez-Solano L, Macia MD, Fajardo A, et al. Chronic *Pseudomonas aeruginosa* infection in chronic obstructive pulmonary disease. *Clin Infect Dis.* 2008;47:1526-33.

44. Sutherland ER, Crapo JD, Bowler RP. N-acetylcysteine and exacerbations of chronic obstructive pulmonary disease. *COPD.* 2006;3:195-202.

45. Murio C, Soler X, Perez M, et al. Acute exacerbation of chronic obstructive pulmonary disease in primary care setting in Spain: the EPOCAP study. *Ther Adv Respir Dis.* 2010; 4:215-23.

46. Effing T, Monninkhof EM, van der Valk PD, et al. Self-management education for patients with chronic obstructive pulmonary disease. *Cochrane Database Syst Rev.* 2007;(4):CD002990.

47. Calverley P, Pauwels Dagger R, Lofdahl CG, et al. Relationship between respiratory symptoms and medical treatment in exacerbations of COPD. *Eur Respir J.* 2005;26: 406-13.

48. Coxson HO, Quiney B, Sin DD, et al. Airway wall thickness assessed using computed tomography and optical coherence tomography. *Am J Respir Crit Care Med.* 2008;177: 1201-6.

Acute Exacerbations of Asthma

Sonia Bains

INTRODUCTION

Asthma exacerbations are responsible for most of the morbidity and mortality associated with asthma, and account for more than 80% of direct costs of asthma.[1] Although exacerbations are more frequent in severe asthmatics, even with excellent adherence to aggressive guidelines-based therapy, up to 42% of adolescents experience at least one exacerbation annually.[2]

DEFINITION

An acute or subacute episode of progressively worsening shortness of breath, cough, wheezing, and chest tightness, with reduction in expiratory airflow (as measured by a drop in forced expiratory volume in 1 second (FEV_1) or peak expiratory flow rate (PEFR)).[3] There is no clear consensus definition; clinical trials usually define an exacerbation by documenting the need for systemic corticosteroids, hospital admission, or emergency department (ED) treatment.[4] Asthma exacerbations can be classified as mild, moderate, severe, and life-threatening. Table 2-1 reviews the signs, symptoms, PEFR, and FEV_1 to classify the severity of an attack. It also suggests appropriate actions to be taken by the patient with or without physician.

EPIDEMIOLOGY

The prevalence of asthma among adults has increased by 75% between 1980 and 1994.[5] Boys experience more cxacerbations than girls before puberty, resulting in more hospitalization and ED visits. At puberty, the sex difference reverses; and women are twice as likely as men to be hospitalized for acute asthma. Duration of hospitalization tends to be longer, and readmission is also more common in women as compared to men.[6] There is a 3- to 4-fold increase in hospitalizations and ED visits for asthma, beginning in mid-August, reaching a peak around 2 weeks after school return in children 5–15 years of age (the September epidemic).[7] In patients over the age of 50 years, a peak in hospitalizations and ED visits is observed between December and January.[8] Children and adolescents have the lowest mortality rate (0.02%) and the elderly have the highest mortality rate from asthma (1.9% for ages

Table 2-1	Classification of Asthma Exacerbation Severity		
Severity	*Signs and symptoms*	*PEFR or FEV$_1$ (% of personal best or % predicted)*	*Recommended action/ clinical course*
Mild	Symptoms only with activity Prompt relief with SABA	≥ 70	Use SABA q 4–6 hours until resolved If symptoms persist beyond 24 hours, call physician's office Oral steroid course may be required
Moderate	Symptoms limit activity Relief with frequent SABA	40–69	Use SABA q15 minutes See your physician or go to ED Oral steroid course is required, may take 1–2 days for resolution
Severe	Symptoms at rest Partial relief with SABA Possible cyanosis	< 40	Use SABA q15 minutes Proceed to ED May require hospitalization Oral steroids required, may take more than 3 days for resolution Adjunct therapies may be helpful
Life-threatening	Inability to speak in complete sentences, drowsy or confused Minimal/no relief from SABA	< 25	Proceed to ED Requires hospitalization, possibly to ICU Requires IV steroids Adjunct therapies may be helpful

Adapted from Expert Panel Report 3 (EPR-3). Guidelines for the diagnosis and management of asthma-summary report 2007. *J Allergy Clin Immunol.* 2007;120:S94-138.

> 75).[9] Race and ethnicity also play a major role in risk of asthma exacerbation. African Americans and Hispanic patients, especially Puerto Ricans, are at a higher risk than Caucasians to be admitted to the hospital for an asthma exacerbation.[10] Mortality is higher in African Americans, followed by Hispanics, and then Caucasians.[10] This may be due to differences in access to healthcare, poor preventive management and delays in seeking medical attention.

Exacerbation-prone Phenotype

While some patients have rare and intermittent exacerbations, a subset of asthmatics is exacerbation-prone. This is evident from the fact that 73% of patients, presenting to an ED for acute asthma, report at least one ED visit related to asthma in the past year, and 21% report six or more visits.[11] Non-white race, medicaid or no insurance, and markers of asthma severity have been identified as risk factors for increased frequency of ED visits. Ten Brinke et al. reported that factors associated with frequent asthma exacerbations (n = 136) included psychological dysfunction (OR 10.8); recurrent respiratory infections (OR 6.9); gastroesophageal reflux disease (OR 4.9); severe rhinosinusitis (OR 3.7); and obstructive sleep apnea (OR 3.4). Severe chronic sinus disease and psychological dysfunction were the only independently associated risk factors.[12] Smoking has been reported to be the most powerful independent modifiable risk factor for multiple severe exacerbations. Intrinsic host defects may also predispose to frequent exacerbations including a defective antiviral response by airway epithelial cells and macrophages. Two polymorphisms in the IL-4 receptor gene have also been associated with an increased risk of severe exacerbations and lower lung function in two independent cohorts.[9]

Subgroup at Risk for Near Fatal Asthma (NFA)

A subgroup of asthmatics experiences severe exacerbations resulting in respiratory failure, requiring ICU admission, and mechanical ventilation. This subgroup differs from asthmatics of all severity groups in two major respects, medication nonadherence and lower corticosteroid use.[13] Interestingly, the NFA group is more comparable to mild-moderate asthmatics rather than severe asthmatics, with respect to clinical and inflammatory parameters. Other studies have confirmed that the NFA group is not distinguished by lung function, airway hyperresponsiveness, smoking status, ethnicity, and prevalence of atopy.[14] This comprises a key subgroup because better interventions for education, adherence, and use of inhaled corticosteroids might reduce the incidence of near-fatal events. A history of serious asthma exacerbations should be elicited, as it adds to the ability of other clinical tools, such as spirometry and asthma control test questionnaire, to predict the future clinical course. Factors predicting increased risk of asthma-related death are enlisted in table 2-2.

CAUSES OF ASTHMA EXACERBATION

The precipitants of acute asthma exacerbation include viruses, allergens (dust mite, pollen, and animal dander), occupational exposures (grains, flours, cleaning agents, metals, irritants, and woods), hormones (menstrual asthma), drugs (aspirin, nonsteroidal anti-inflammatory drugs, beta blockers), concomitant diseases (chronic sinusitis), exercise, psychological stress, air pollutants, and medication nonadherence. Rhinovirus is the most common cause of asthma exacerbation, both in adults and children.[15,16] Other infectious causes include coronavirus, influenza virus, parainfluenza virus, respiratory syncytial virus, *Chlamydia pneumoniae*, and *Mycoplasma pneumoniae*. Lack of anti-inflammatory therapy is a key factor

Table 2-2	Subgroup At-risk for Asthma-related Death
Previous severe exacerbation (requiring ICU admission or intubation)	
More than or equal to two hospitalizations or more than three ED visits in the past year	
Hospitalization or ED visit in the past month	
Use of more than two canisters of short-acting beta agonist per month	
Poor perception of symptoms	
Lack of a written asthma action plan	
Sensitivity to *Alternaria*	
Low socioeconomic status or inner city residence	
Illicit drug use	
Psychosocial dysfunction or psychiatric disease	
Comorbidities: Other lung disease or cardiovascular disease.	

in allowing viral associated worsening.[17] A synergistic interaction is likely to exist between allergic sensitization and viral respiratory infection, resulting in asthma exacerbation. Green et al. showed the odds of asthma exacerbation due to allergen exposure increased from 2.3 to 8.4, when combined with a viral infection.[18] There is an increased risk of exacerbation in asthmatic children and young adults, homozygous for the Arg 16 variant of the Arg 16 Gly beta-2-adrenergic receptor polymorphism.[19]

PREVENTION OF ASTHMA EXACERBATION: THE BEST CURE

Asthma control can be monitored in two domains: impairment and risk.

Impairment is an evaluation of the current degree of control of symptoms and lung function. An increased frequency of symptoms and a decline in FEV_1 indicate that the patient may be at increased risk of an exacerbation.[20]

The risk domain includes criteria that deal with future events which the treatment program aims to prevent, including reduction in the frequency and severity of exacerbations. Presence of comorbidities that may exacerbate asthma (e.g., sinusitis) should be evaluated (Figure 2-1).

Avoidance of allergens, eliminating environmental tobacco smoke exposure, and smoking cessation are most beneficial measures in preventing exacerbations. Emphasis on daily controller therapy is of utmost importance. The GOAL (gaining optimal asthma control) study clearly showed that exacerbations could be reduced in the majority of patients by increasing daily doses of fluticasone and salmeterol until the patient becomes symptom free.[21] The combination of formoterol and budesonide is used both as maintenance and reliever therapies rather than maintenance therapy alone has also shown the potential to reduce exacerbations.[8] Inhaled corticosteroids (ICS) are the most effective strategy, reducing asthma exacerbations by 55%, compared to placebo or short-acting beta agonists alone. Long-acting beta agonists

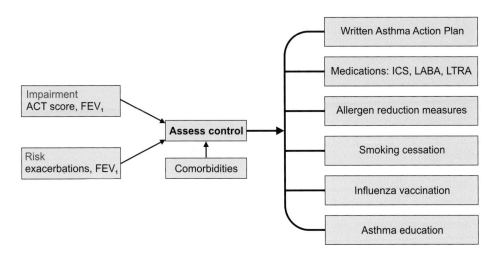

Figure 2-1 Prevention of asthma exacerbation, the best cure. Assess asthma control based upon current level of impairment and future risk of exacerbation. Assess for presence of comorbidities that may exacerbate asthma. Management is based upon measures to reduce the risk of asthma exacerbation which include providing the patient with a written asthma action plan, initiating or continuing controller medications, education about allergen reduction measures, smoking cessation, the importance of influenza vaccination in every fall and lastly focused asthma education. ACT, asthma control test; ICS, inhaled corticosteroids; LABA, long-acting beta agonists; LTRA, leukotriene receptor antagonists.

(LABA) reduce exacerbations by 25% as compared to placebo and also reduce further exacerbations by 26% when added to ICS. Leukotriene modifiers reduce exacerbations by as much as 41%, when compared to placebo. However, they are inferior to ICS in reducing exacerbations and less effective than a LABA as add-on therapy for those already taking ICS. Omalizumab is a humanized monoclonal antibody to IgE that has been shown to reduce exacerbations by approximately 50% even in patients taking high doses of ICS.[9] Annual influenza immunization 4–6 weeks before "flu" season as well as H1N1 immunization can reduce acute asthma cases caused by these common triggers. Influenza vaccination can be safely given to asthmatics during an exacerbation.

Identifying patients with risk factors for near-fatal or fatal asthma is paramount in preventing fatalities and exacerbations. A written asthma action plan is crucial to reduce office or ED visits for acute asthma. An action plan should include symptoms and objective measures, such as PEFR, to aid in early recognition of exacerbation and its severity. Simple and clear medication instructions, physician's contact numbers, and emergency care steps must be included. The asthma action plan, various medications, inhaler technique, and PEFR measurements should be reviewed with the patient at each office visit. Exhaled nitric oxide (a biomarker of inflammation), responsiveness to methacholine challenge, and sputum eosinophil counts have been used to guide asthma management. In each case, this additional monitoring has resulted in fewer exacerbations.[8]

MANAGEMENT OF ACUTE EXACERBATION

The goals of managing an asthma exacerbation are prompt recognition, rapid reversal of airflow obstruction, avoidance of relapses, and prevention of future episodes.

Home Management

All patients diagnosed with asthma should have a written asthma action plan. Parents or caregivers should be educated to recognize common triggers of asthma including viral upper respiratory infections with or without allergens. If exposed, they should remove themselves from that environment and start daily and as needed PEFR monitoring to identify a downward trend, which may precede frank symptoms. Persistent cough, chest tightness, shortness of breath or wheeze, and PEFR of less than 80% of personal best should prompt treatment with 2–6 puffs of a short-acting beta agonist (SABA) metered-dose inhaler (MDI) with spacer or a single nebulized bronchodilator treatment. If symptoms persist 20 minutes after the treatment or worsen, or if PEFR remains less than 80% of personal best, patients should repeat the treatment and call their physician. Patients should be provided with a 24-hour telephone number and encouraged to contact their physician. If symptoms improve and do not recur, no further treatment is required. A few indications, for initiating a 3- to 10-day oral corticosteroid burst at home for symptomatic patients with PEFR more than 50% but less than 80% personal best, include recurrent symptoms requiring every 4–6-hourly bronchodilator treatments, nocturnal awakenings with asthma symptoms, and prolonged symptoms or limitation of activities. Patients with PEFR less than 50% of personal best marked wheezing or shortness of breath should continue to take nebulized bronchodilator therapy, initiate oral corticosteroids, and proceed to the ED.

Outpatient Management (Physician's Office)

The first and most crucial step is to differentiate patients with impending respiratory failure from all others. All patients must be aggressively treated with bronchodilators, oxygen and oral corticosteroids during the first hour to determine their disposition. Patients who have not shown improvement after initial albuterol treatment should receive albuterol plus ipratropium. Oral corticosteroids should be administered within the first hour. If there is no response after three bronchodilator treatments, the patient will likely need to be hospitalized and should be transferred to the ED.

MANAGING ASTHMA EXACERBATION IN THE ED: A SUMMARY OF THE NATIONAL ASTHMA EDUCATION AND PREVENTION PROGRAM EXPERT PANEL REPORT-3 (NAEPP EPR-3) GUIDELINES[3]

Initial Assessment

Classifying the Severity of Asthma Exacerbations

The primary determinant of the severity of an exacerbation is the percent predicted FEV_1 or percent of personal best PEFR, as presented in the new EPR-3 guidelines. Exacerbation severity determines treatment. Mild exacerbations can usually be treated at home, but more severe exacerbations require treatment and monitoring in the ED; and in more serious cases, hospital admission. All patients presenting to the ED should undergo a focused evaluation including history, physical examination and assessment of lung function (Figure 2-2).

Focused History

- Time of onset of symptoms
- Cause of exacerbation
- Severity of symptoms
- Response to any treatment given before admission to the ED
- Number of previous ED visits and hospital admissions, especially in the previous year
- History of intubation
- Comorbidities
- Current medications and time of last dose of asthma medications.

Physical Examination

- Vital signs
- Level of alertness
- Fluid status
- Signs of respiratory distress
- Exclude vocal cord dysfunction and other causes of upper airway obstruction; clues include dysphonia, inspiratory stridor, monophonic wheezing that is loudest over the central airway, normal $PaCO_2$ and complete resolution of airflow obstruction with intubation.

Lung Function

- Assessment of lung function should be done in all patients over 5 years of age by measuring FEV_1 or PEFR
- It should be done at presentation and then repeated at 30–60 minutes after initial treatment; useful in categorizing the severity of exacerbation
- Pulse oximetry.

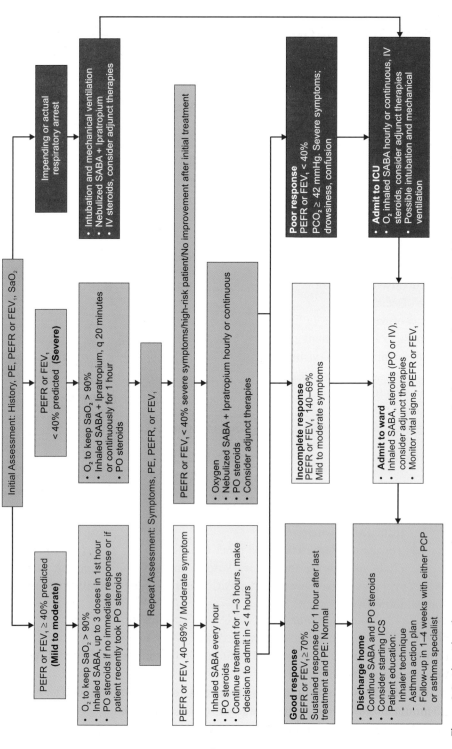

Figure 2-2 Algorithm for emergency department management of asthma exacerbation. *Adapted from* Expert Panel Report 3 (EPR-3). Guidelines for the diagnosis and management of asthma-summary report 2007. *J Allergy Clin Immunol.* 2007;120:S94-138.

Laboratory Studies

- Mostly, patients require none
- Laboratory studies may be used to detect respiratory failure, theophylline toxicity or complications such as pneumonia
- An arterial blood gas analysis can be done to evaluate $PaCO_2$
- Complete blood count (CBC) may be appropriate in patients with fever and purulent sputum
- Chest radiograph is not routinely required, except in patients suspected of having congestive heart failure, pneumothorax, pneumomediastinum, or pneumonia.

Emergency Department Management

In general, primary treatments (i.e., oxygen, inhaled beta-2 agonists, and systemic corticosteroids) are the same for all asthma exacerbations, but the dose and frequency of administration along with the frequency of patient monitoring depend on the severity of the asthma exacerbation. The SaO_2 should be maintained more than 90%, and more than 95% in pregnant patients and patients with concomitant heart disease.[22] Three treatments of inhaled beta-2 agonists administered every 20–30 minutes should be tried initially, as this is the most effective means of acutely reversing airflow obstruction.[23] About 60–70% of patients will respond sufficiently to the initial three doses to be discharged.[23] In patients with severe exacerbations (i.e., PEFR < 40%), continuous administration of beta-2 agonists may be more effective than intermittent dosing.[24] Systemic corticosteroids are recommended for most of the patients because they speed the resolution of airflow obstruction and reduce the rate of post-ED relapse.[25] Oral steroids should be administered to all patients with moderate-to-severe exacerbations and to those who do not respond to initial beta-2 agonist therapy.[22] Oral steroids reduce the likelihood of hospitalization, if started early in patients with moderate-to-severe exacerbations.[25] Oral prednisone has been shown to have effects equivalent to that of intravenous methylprednisolone and thus, oral steroids should be administered.[3] Ipratropium bromide should be added to beta-2 agonist therapy to increase bronchodilation. The combination of a beta-2 agonist and inhaled ipratropium bromide has been shown to reduce hospitalizations, particularly in patients with severe airflow obstruction.[26,27] The expert panel does not recommend use of methylxanthines, chest physiotherapy, mucolytics or sedation. Although most acute wheezing episodes are accompanied by fever, antibiotics are generally not necessary, as most episodes are viral rather than bacterial (Figure 2-2).

All patients should be assessed within 60–90 minutes after initiation of therapy which is after three doses of inhaled bronchodilator treatment. Response to treatment in the ED is a better predictor of the need for hospitalization than the severity of an exacerbation at the time of presentation.[28] All repeated assessments should include the patient's subjective response to treatment, physical examination, FEV_1 or PEFR (SaO_2, and arterial blood gas analysis, if indicated). Patients who do not show improvement after three bronchodilator treatments are unlikely to improve with more treatments in the ED and should be considered for hospitalization. Patients who show slow but steady improvement can be treated longer in the ED for 1–3 hours. Those who get worse in the course of therapy require an arterial blood gas analysis. Indications for admission to the hospital are enlisted in tables 2-3 and 2-4.

Patient Discharge

Patients who demonstrate a rapid response to treatment should be observed for 30–60 minutes after the most recent dose of bronchodilator therapy to ensure stability of response before discharge to home. In general, patients can be discharged if FEV_1 or PEFR is > 70% predicted or personal best and symptoms are minimal or absent. Patients treated with corticosteroids should be discharged on 3- to 10-day course of oral steroids.

Anti-inflammatory Treatment after Discharge to Home from the ED

Anti-inflammatory therapy with systemic corticosteroids is a cornerstone of the management of patients with acute asthma.[3,29] Unfortunately, up to one-third of patients relapse within the first 3–4 weeks after ED discharge.[30,31] Krishnan et al. conducted a systematic review of the literature (N = 599) and determined that:

Table 2-3	Indications for Hospitalization
FEV_1 or PEFR < 60% of personal best despite treatment
SaO_2 < 90% on RA
Multiple recent asthma-related visits to the ED or physician's office
Recent hospitalization for asthma
History of ICU admission or intubation for asthma
Prolonged duration of symptoms
Multiple triggers
Poor access to medications and medical follow-up
Lack of understanding of the disease and its management
Psychiatric or psychosocial conditions.

Table 2-4	Indications for ICU Admission
FEV_1 < 30% with marked respiratory distress
Worsening symptoms despite treatment
$PaCO_2$ > 42 mmHg with or without PaO_2 < 60 mmHg
Impending respiratory failure
High-risk status or history of near-fatal asthma.

(i) intramuscular corticosteroids are as effective as oral corticosteroid regimens in preventing relapse; (ii) in those (N = 269) with mild-to-moderate acute asthma, inhaled corticosteroids and oral corticosteroids are similarly effective in preventing relapse; (iii) a nonsignificant trend suggested that combination therapy with inhaled and oral corticosteroids might be more effective than oral corticosteroids alone (n = 912); and (iv) additional studies are required to examine the safety and efficacy of initiating macrolide antibiotics and leukotriene modifiers after an episode of acute asthma.[32] Nonadherence to oral corticosteroid treatment is common even immediately after ED or hospital discharge;[33,34] and therefore, intramuscular steroids may be preferable in patients at risk of noncompliance.

Observational studies suggest that inhaled corticosteroids reduce acute asthma relapse by about 50%.[35-37] Unfortunately, a number of studies have documented low rates of inhaled corticosteroid prescription at ED discharge after acute asthma (16–24%).[38-40] It is recommended by the EPR-3 to discharge patients with daily inhaled corticosteroids (in addition to oral corticosteroids), when there is evidence of persistent asthma between episodes of acute asthma and in patients with an exacerbation in the prior 12 months.[3] It must be kept in mind, however, that inhaled steroids are most costly and difficult for patients to use compared to oral corticosteroids. As poor inhaler technique is common in patients who are present with acute asthma, all patients prescribed ICS should receive adequate training before ED discharge.[41-43]

Education of the Asthmatic Patient in the ED

Focused patient education should occur including general asthma education, review of inhaler technique, a simple written asthma discharge plan and referral for follow-up within 1 week with either primary care physician (PCP) or an asthma specialist. Following an ED visit for acute asthma, rates of follow-up with primary care providers are often low.[44] Effective and timely outpatient care of asthma can prevent adverse asthma outcomes, specifically ED visits and hospitalizations.[45,46] Scahtz et al. performed a systematic review of the literature to identify strategies to reduce the rate of subsequent exacerbations. Their findings are summarized in table 2-5.[47]

Impending Respiratory Failure

Early recognition and treatment are essential, as respiratory failure can progress rapidly and is difficult to reverse. Signs include an inability to speak, altered mental status, intercostal retraction, worsening fatigue and a $PaCO_2$ of 42 mmHg or greater.

Noninvasive Positive Pressure Ventilation (NPPV)

There are two principal forms, continuous positive airway pressure (CPAP) and bilevel positive airway pressure (BiPAP). Both have been used as an alternative to intubation

Table 2-5	What Improves Outcomes after Asthma Exacerbation?
Classify asthma severity according to 2007 NAEPP guideline	
Discharge on a 3- to 10-day course of oral steroids or administer IM steroid injection in ED	
Provide a simple, written asthma discharge plan	
Start ICS if the patient has persistent asthma or has had an exacerbation in the prior 12 months	
Instruct on inhaler technique	
Schedule a follow-up appointment with the PCP (for mild asthmatics) and with asthma specialist for moderate and severe persistent asthma	
Follow-up appointment should be within 1 week of the ED visit.	

in a variety of respiratory conditions, avoiding the complications associated with endotracheal intubation.[48] Low-level CPAP offsets the detrimental effects of auto-positive end-expiratory pressure (auto-PEEP), which are caused by gas trapped in alveoli at end expiration and, decreases inspiratory work of breathing.[49] BiPAP generally improves tidal volume in proportion to the pressure applied.[50] Nowak et al. performed a systematic review of the literature which suggests that NPPV might be a useful adjunct in the treatment of severe asthma exacerbations. However, data from randomized, prospective, controlled trials are minimal. Although no definitive conclusion regarding the role of NPPV in the treatment of acute severe asthma can be made, the authors suggest following points:

- A trial of NPPV before intubation and mechanical ventilation should be considered in patients who can cooperate with and tolerate therapy. It should only be used in a closely-monitored setting with trained personnel and the ability to immediately intubate the patient, if needed
- Pending additional data, specific settings should follow the protocol set forth in the article by Soroksky et al.[51]

Given the minimal complications reported to date with NPPV use in patients with an asthma exacerbation and the potential ability to avoid intubation and mechanical ventilation, this approach seems reasonable pending further clinical trials.[52]

Intubation and Mechanical Ventilation of the Asthmatic Patient in Respiratory Failure

Prevention of Intubation

This is an important goal because mortality ranges from 10 to 20% in patients with acute asthma who require intubation.[53] Most asthmatics are able to be treated without intubation.[54,55] Patients typically respond to first and second-line therapies; however, some may not respond, in which case alternative therapies may be used such as heliox, ketamine, glucagon, leukotriene inhibitors, nebulized clonidine, nitroglycerin, nebulized calcium channel blockers, nebulized lidocaine, and external chest compression.[56] Intravenous magnesium may be considered in those with life-threatening exacerbations and attacks that remain severe after one hour of intensive conventional treatment.[57] Heliox-driven albuterol nebulization can also be considered in these patients to decrease the work of breathing.[58] Intravenous beta-2 agonist administration is a largely unapproved treatment and the Expert Panel does not recommend its use in acute asthma exacerbation because of the danger of myocardial toxicity.

Criteria for Intubation

There are four indications for intubation: cardiac arrest, respiratory arrest, physical exhaustion, and altered sensorium (lethargy or agitation). Increasing $PaCO_2$ alone is not an indication for intubation. It is only indicated, if $PaCO_2$ is increasing by > 5 mmHg/hour or is greater than 55–70 mmHg despite medical management and associated with a change in mental status.[59] Other indications include a pH less than 7.20 or SaO_2 less than 60 mmHg on 100% oxygen. It should be done immediately in a patient presenting with apnea or coma. Semi-elective intubation should be performed prior to respiratory arrest.

Intubation Technique

There are four choices of technique, each with its own benefits and risks: nasotracheal intubation; awake orotracheal intubation; orotracheal intubation with sedation; orotracheal intubation with sedation and neuromuscular blockade. In general, orotracheal intubation with sedation and neuromuscular blockade is preferred for asthmatic patients in critical respiratory distress. Nasotracheal intubation may potentially be complicated by nasal polyps and sinus disease, commonly found in patients with asthma. Pretreatment with bronchodilators may reduce airway bronchospasm associated with tracheal intubation.

Recommendations for Appropriate Ventilator Settings

When an asthmatic patient is ventilated, severe hyperinflation can result from breath stacking, placing the patient at risk for hypotension and barotrauma.[60] It is essential to recognize, measure, and control hyperinflation and auto-PEEP to ensure a good outcome in the intubated asthmatic patient. Auto-PEEP occurs when diminished expiratory flow causes incomplete emptying of alveolar gas. As end-expiratory lung volume increases, so does end-inspiratory lung volume for a given tidal volume, predisposing the patient to lung hyperinflation.[61] There are three ventilator strategies that can be used to reduce hyperinflation and auto-PEEP in the intubated asthmatic patient: reduction of the respiratory rate, reduction of tidal volume, and shortening of inspiration by increasing inspiratory flow to allow greater time for exhalation with each respiratory cycle. Changes in the respiratory rate have the greatest effect on hyperinflation and auto-PEEP. In most patients, a peak inspiratory flow of 60 L/minute (constant flow) or 80–90 L/minute (decelerating flow) is reasonable during the initial set up of the ventilator. Tidal volume should be set at 7–8 mL/kg (ideal body weight). Respiratory rate should be set at 10 breaths/minute and fraction of inspired oxygen at 1.0.[56] If one is unable to reduce the respiratory rate enough for reduction of hyperinflation and auto-PEEP to acceptable levels (10–15 cmH$_2$O), inspiratory time can be shortened to allow a longer time for exhalation per respiratory cycle. This can be achieved by increasing the inspiratory flow rate. Reduction of tidal volume is appropriate; however, it is limited by its progressive effect on dead-space fraction. Decreasing respiratory rate can result in hypercapnia; fortunately, this is usually well-tolerated, even with PaCO$_2$ as high as 90 mmHg. In selected critically-ill patients, it may be safer to accept hypercapnia than to overventilate to a normal PaCO$_2$ at the cost of hyperinflation. An acceptable level of hypercapnia and acidosis is a pH as low as 7.15 and a PaCO$_2$ of up to 80 mmHg. Anoxic brain injury and myocardial dysfunction are contraindications to permissive hypercapnia because of the potential for hypercapnia to dilate cerebral vessels, constrict pulmonary vessels and decrease myocardial contractility.[62]

Determining the severity of lung, hyperinflation is central to assessing patients and adjusting ventilator settings. In common practice, two relatively easy to measure pressures are used as surrogate markers of lung inflation; auto-PEEP and plateau pressure (Pplat). Auto-PEEP is an estimate of the lowest average alveolar pressure achieved during the respiratory cycle. Pplat (or lung distention pressure) estimates average end-inspiratory alveolar pressure. Accurate measurements of Pplat and auto-PEEP require patient-ventilator synchrony and absence of patient effort. Paralysis is generally not required. Unfortunately, neither auto-PEEP nor Pplat has been validated as a predictor of complications of mechanical ventilation. Still, many experts agree that complications are rare when Pplat is less than 30 cmH$_2$O and auto-PEEP is less than 15 cmH$_2$O.[56]

Management in the Immediate Post-intubation Period

Endotracheal tube placement should be verified with a carbon dioxide detector, adequate oximeter readings and chest radiography. Post-intubation sedation should be provided with a benzodiazepine which improves patient's comfort, decreases oxygen consumption and carbon dioxide production, and allows synchronism between the patient and the ventilator.[63] Neuromuscular blockade should be limited, when possible, to less than 24 hours to avoid an associated myopathy, as deep sedation is all that is required by that time.[61] Heliox, a mixture of oxygen and helium, decreases airway resistance by reducing airflow turbulence in the bronchial passages. The results of studies on the benefits of heliox are conflicting, but there might be some benefit to its use in patients before intubation as a means of avoiding intubation. There is currently insufficient evidence to support the use of heliox in intubated patients.[56]

Medical Management of Asthma in the Intubated Patient

As bronchospasm continues after intubation, inhaled bronchodilators and systemic corticosteroids should be continued.[61] Systemic corticosteroids are the gold standard of treatment. Manser et al. conducted a systematic review of the literature and determined that 40 mg every 6 hours of methylprednisolone (or equivalent) is appropriate and higher doses do not appear to be more efficacious.[64] Beta agonists are also indicated either nebulized or inhaled.[65] The clinical benefits of intravenous theophylline in intubated patients are unknown, but outcomes in hospitalized asthmatic patients do not appear to improve.[3]

Prevention and Treatment of Complications

- *Intubation-induced bronchospasm:* Pretreatment with bronchodilators is useful in decreasing and preventing this complication of intubation.[66]
- *Persistent hypoxemia:* This suggests a complication of mechanical ventilation such as right mainstem intubation, pneumothorax, endotracheal tube displacement, endotracheal tube blockage, leakage of air around the endotracheal tube, gastric distention, mechanical malfunction of the ventilator apparatus, aspiration, progressive bronchospasm, or pneumonia or other lung disease. These all must be addressed individually as appropriate.
- *Hypotension:* This is another frequently encountered complication during mechanical ventilation. In critical hypotension (defined as a decrease in systolic blood pressure to < 90 mmHg or a reduction of > 40 mmHg from baseline value), a trial of hypopnea (2–3 breaths/minute) or apnea in a preoxygenated patient for 30–60 seconds can be both diagnostic and therapeutic for lung hyperinflation as a cause of hypotension. Consider pneumothorax, especially if there is a tracheal shift with unilateral breath sounds or subcutaneous emphysema and no response to a trial of apnea or hypopnea. Tension pneumothorax is a clinical diagnosis. If lung examination suggests this complication, proceed with a needle thoracostomy followed by a chest tube thoracostomy. Auto-PEEP and Pplat should be measured and reduction measures should be applied. Other causes, such as myocardial infarction and sepsis, must be excluded. Critical hypotension, for which a reversible cause cannot be immediately found, is an indication for epinephrine.
- *Cardiac arrest:* This can be a result of critical lung hyperinflation. A trial of apnea or hypopnea for not more than 30–60 seconds, external chest compressions, volume challenge and epinephrine are indicated for cardiac arrest presenting as pulseless electrical activity. If tension pneumothorax is suspected, proceed as above. Other causes may include hypoxemia, acidemia, electrolyte abnormalities (including lethal hyperkalemia, if succinylcholine was used for intubation of

CASE STUDY

A 33-year-old African-American male with past medical history of severe persistent asthma presents to the emergency department (ED) with worsening shortness of breath, coughing, chest tightness and wheezing for the past four days, with multiple nocturnal awakenings due to these symptoms. He reports a history of three ED visits in the last 12 months due to asthma exacerbations. Currently, he has no signs of significant respiratory distress. On examination, the patient is mildly tachypneic at rest, able to speak in complete sentences, and has loud bilateral expiratory wheezing on auscultation.

1. *What is the most appropriate initial step in this patient's management?*
   The appropriate initial step is to check pulse oximetry, provide oxygen, and administer inhaled albuterol via MDI. This can be repeated every 20 minutes for up to three treatments.
2. *What initial diagnostic studies should be obtained for a patient who presents to the ED with an acute asthma exacerbation?*
   Most patients require none; however, they may be done to detect respiratory failure (an arterial blood gas to evaluate $PaCO_2$), theophylline toxicity, or complications such as pneumonia (complete blood count with differential may be appropriate in patients with fever and purulent sputum). A chest radiograph is not routinely required, except in patients suspected of having congestive heart failure, pneumothorax, pneumomediastinum, or pneumonia.
3. *After an hour of appropriate treatments, the patient's status is reassessed. The patient's personal best peak flow is 400 L/min, and his current best peak flow rate is 200 L/min. The patient appears to be in no respiratory distress and his oxygen saturation is 96% on 2 L via nasal cannula. He has some mild expiratory wheezes bilaterally. How would you classify this patient's exacerbation using the current NHLBI definition?*
   The patient is having an asthma exacerbation of moderate severity. This is based upon a peak expiratory flow rate of 50 percent of personal best. An exacerbation is classified according to the NHLBI as being of moderate severity, if the PEFR is between 40% and 69% of personal best.
4. *What is the next best step in the management of this patient?*
   The next best step is to administer oral corticosteroids and continue treatment with albuterol via MDI every hour in the ED. This treatment should be continued for the next 1–4 hours and if there is inadequate response, then a decision to admit should be made within that time period. An inadequate response is indicated by lack of sustained benefit from albuterol past an hour and inability to increase PEFR above 70%. Systemic corticosteroids reduce the likelihood of hospitalization if started early and the rate of post-ED relapse.
5. *Is this patient at increased risk of asthma-related death?*
   This patient is at elevated risk of asthma-related death given his history of three ED visits in the past year due to asthma exacerbations.

a patient with respiratory acidosis) and endotracheal tube displacement or blockage. Use of illicit drugs, such as heroin or cocaine, should also be considered.

- *Barotrauma:* Increased morbidity and mortality are associated with barotrauma. Parameters to detect barotrauma including airway pressure, PEEP, tidal volume are controversial and volume at end expiration should be closely monitored to detect barotrauma.

- *Myopathy:* Behbehani et al. reported a high incidence of acute myopathy when neuromuscular blocking agents were used for near-fatal asthma, but corticosteroids were not independently associated with myopathy in their study.[67]

- *Extubation:* Weaning and extubation criteria have not been validated for patients with acute asthma. One approach is to perform a spontaneous breathing trial in an awake patient; once $PaCO_2$ normalizes, airway resistance is less than 20 cmH_2O, auto-PEEP is less than 10 cmH_2O and there is no evidence of neuromuscular weakness. Extubation should proceed in a timely manner to avoid complications. After extubation, observation in an ICU is recommended for an additional 12–24 hours.[56]

REFERENCES

1. Rodrigo GJ, Rodrigo C, Hall JB. Acute asthma in adults: a review. *Chest.* 2004;125:1081-102.
2. Szefler SJ, et al. Management of asthma based on exhaled nitric oxide in addition to guideline-based treatment for inner-city adolescents and young adults: a randomised controlled trial. *Lancet.* 2008;372:1065-72.
3. Expert Panel Report 3 (EPR-3). Guidelines for the diagnosis and management of asthma-summary report 2007. *J Allergy Clin Immunol.* 2007;120:S94-138.
4. O'Byrne PM, et al. Low dose inhaled budesonide and formoterol in mild persistent asthma: the OPTIMA randomized trial. *Am J Respir Crit Care Med.* 2001;164:1392-7.
5. Mannino DM, et al. Surveillance for asthma—United States, 1960-1995. *MMWR CDC Surveill Summ.* 1998;47:1-27.
6. Schatz M, Clark S, Camargo CA. Sex differences in the presentation and course of asthma hospitalizations. *Chest.* 2006;129:50-5.
7. Sears MR, Johnston NW. Understanding the September asthma epidemic. *J Allergy Clin Immunol.* 2007;120:526-9.
8. Sears MR. Epidemiology of asthma exacerbations. *J Allergy Clin Immunol.* 2008;122: 662-8; quiz 669-70.
9. Dougherty RH, Fahy JV. Acute exacerbations of asthma: epidemiology, biology and the exacerbation-prone phenotype. *Clin Exp Allergy.* 2009;39:193-202.
10. Krishnan V, et al. Mortality in patients hospitalized for asthma exacerbations in the United States. *Am J Respir Crit Care Med.* 2006;174:633-8.
11. Griswold SK, et al. Asthma exacerbations in North American adults: who are the "frequent fliers" in the emergency department? *Chest.* 2005;127:1579-86.
12. Ten Brinke A, et al. Risk factors of frequent exacerbations in difficult-to-treat asthma. *Eur Respir J.* 2005;26:812-8.
13. Romagnoli M, et al. Near-fatal asthma phenotype in the ENFUMOSA Cohort. *Clin Exp Allergy.* 2007;37:552-7.

14. Alvarez GG, et al. A systematic review of risk factors associated with near-fatal and fatal asthma. *Can Respir J.* 2005;12:265-70.
15. Atmar RL, et al. Respiratory tract viral infections in inner-city asthmatic adults. *Arch Intern Med.* 1998;158:2453-9.
16. Heymann PW, et al. Viral infections in relation to age, atopy, and season of admission among children hospitalized for wheezing. *J Allergy Clin Immunol.* 2004;114:239-47.
17. Johnston NW, et al. The September epidemic of asthma exacerbations in children: a search for etiology. *J Allergy Clin Immunol.* 2005;115:132-8.
18. Green RM, et al. Synergism between allergens and viruses and risk of hospital admission with asthma: case-control study. *BMJ.* 2002;324:763.
19. Basu K, et al. Adrenergic beta(2)-receptor genotype predisposes to exacerbations in steroid-treated asthmatic patients taking frequent albuterol or salmeterol. *J Allergy Clin Immunol.* 2009;124:1188-94.e3.
20. Koga T, et al. Characterization of patients with frequent exacerbation of asthma. *Respir Med.* 2006;100:273-8.
21. Bateman ED, et al. Can guideline-defined asthma control be achieved? The Gaining Optimal Asthma ControL study. *Am J Respir Crit Care Med.* 2004;170:836-44.
22. Camargo CA, Rachelefsky G, Schatz M. Managing asthma exacerbations in the emergency department: summary of the National Asthma Education and Prevention Program Expert Panel Report 3 guidelines for the management of asthma exacerbations. *J Allergy Clin Immunol.* 2009;124:S5-14.
23. Karpel JP, et al. Emergency treatment of acute asthma with albuterol metered-dose inhaler plus holding chamber: how often should treatments be administered? *Chest.* 1997;112:348-56.
24. Camargo CA, Spooner CH, Rowe BH. Continuous versus intermittent beta-agonists in the treatment of acute asthma. *Cochrane Database Syst Rev.* 2003;(4):CD001115.
25. Rowe BH, et al. Corticosteroid therapy for acute asthma. *Respir Med.* 2004;98:275-84.
26. Plotnick LH and Ducharme FM. Combined inhaled anticholinergics and beta2-agonists for initial treatment of acute asthma in children. *Cochrane Database Syst Rev.* 2000;(4):CD000060.
27. Rodrigo GJ, Castro-Rodriguez JA. Anticholinergics in the treatment of children and adults with acute asthma: a systematic review with meta-analysis. *Thorax.* 2005;60:740-6.
28. Kelly AM, Kerr D, Powell C. Is severity assessment after one hour of treatment better for predicting the need for admission in acute asthma? *Respir Med.* 2004;98:777-81.
29. Rowe BH, et al. Corticosteroids for preventing relapse following acute exacerbations of asthma. *Cochrane Database Syst Rev.* 2001;(1):CD000195.
30. Silverman RA, et al. Zafirlukast treatment for acute asthma: evaluation in a randomized, double-blind, multicenter trial. *Chest.* 2004;126:1480-9.
31. Chan JS, et al. Comparison of intramuscular betamethasone and oral prednisone in the prevention of relapse of acute asthma. *Can Respir J.* 2001;8:147-52.
32. Krishnan JA, et al. Anti-inflammatory treatment after discharge home from the emergency department in adults with acute asthma. *J Allergy Clin Immunol.* 2009;124:S29-34.
33. Butler K, Cooper WO. Adherence of pediatric asthma patients with oral corticosteroid prescriptions following pediatric emergency department visit or hospitalization. *Pediatr Emerg Care.* 2004;20:730-5.

34. Krishnan JA, et al. Corticosteroid use after hospital discharge among high-risk adults with asthma. *Am J Respir Crit Care Med.* 2004;170:1281-5.

35. Camargo CA, et al. Association between common asthma therapies and recurrent asthma exacerbations in children enrolled in a state Medicaid plan. *Am J Health Syst Pharm.* 2007;64:1054-61.

36. Smith MJ, Rascati KL, McWilliams BC. Inhaled anti-inflammatory pharmacotherapy and subsequent hospitalizations and emergency department visits among patients with asthma in the Texas Medicaid program. *Ann Allergy Asthma Immunol.* 2004;92:40-6.

37. Sin DD, Man SF. Low-dose inhaled corticosteroid therapy and risk of emergency department visits for asthma. *Arch Intern Med.* 2002;162:1591-5.

38. Salerno EL, et al. Discharge patterns of patients with asthma from the emergency department: a retrospective review. *Conn Med.* 2005;69:621-7.

39. Scarfone RJ, Zorc JJ, Angsuco CJ. Emergency physicians' prescribing of asthma controller medications. *Pediatrics.* 2006;117:821-7.

40. Cydulka RK, et al. Inadequate follow-up controller medications among patients with asthma who visit the emergency department. *Ann Emerg Med.* 2005;46:316-22.

41. Shrestha M, et al. Metered-dose inhaler technique of patients in an urban ED: prevalence of incorrect technique and attempt at education. *Am J Emerg Med.* 1996;14:380-4.

42. Numata Y, et al. Teaching time for metered-dose inhalers in the emergency setting. *Chest.* 2002;122:498-504.

43. Paasche-Orlow MK, et al. Tailored education may reduce health literacy disparities in asthma self-management. *Am J Respir Crit Care Med.* 2005;172:980-6.

44. Leickly FE, et al. Self-reported adherence, management behavior, and barriers to care after an emergency department visit by inner city children with asthma. *Pediatrics.* 1998; 101:E8.

45. Ford ME, et al. Health outcomes among African American and Caucasian adults following a randomized trial of an asthma education program. *Ethn Health.* 1997;2: 329-39.

46. Mayo PH, Richman J, Harris HW. Results of a program to reduce admissions for adult asthma. *Ann Intern Med.* 1990;112:864-71.

47. Schatz M, Rachelefsky G, Krishnan JA. Follow-up after acute asthma episodes: what improves future outcomes? *J Allergy Clin Immunol.* 2009;124:S35-42.

48. Mehta S, Hill NS. Noninvasive ventilation. *Am J Respir Crit Care Med.* 2001;163:540-77.

49. Appendini L, et al. Physiologic effects of positive end-expiratory pressure and mask pressure support during exacerbations of chronic obstructive pulmonary disease. *Am J Respir Crit Care Med.* 1994;149:1069-76.

50. Meyer TJ, Hill NS. Noninvasive positive pressure ventilation to treat respiratory failure. *Ann Intern Med.* 1994;120:760-70.

51. Soroksky A, Stav D, Shpirer I. A pilot prospective, randomized, placebo-controlled trial of bilevel positive airway pressure in acute asthmatic attack. *Chest.* 2003;123:1018-25.

52. Nowak R, Corbridge T, Brenner B. Noninvasive ventilation. *J Allergy Clin Immunol.* 2009;124:S15-8.

53. Shapiro JM. Intensive care management of status asthmaticus. *Chest.* 2001;120:1439-41.

54. Braman SS, Kaemmerlen JT. Intensive care of status asthmaticus. A 10-year experience. *JAMA.* 1990;264:366-8.

55. Mountain RD, et al. Acid-base disturbances in acute asthma. *Chest.* 1990;98:651-5.

56. Brenner B, Corbridge T, Kazzi A. Intubation and mechanical ventilation of the asthmatic patient in respiratory failure. *J Allergy Clin Immunol.* 2009;124:S19-28.

57. Cheuk DK, Chau TC, Lee SL. A meta-analysis on intravenous magnesium sulphate for treating acute asthma. *Arch Dis Child.* 2005;90:74-7.

58. Lee DL, et al. Beneficial effects of albuterol therapy driven by heliox versus by oxygen in severe asthma exacerbation. *Acad Emerg Med.* 2005;12:820-7.

59. Mountain RD, Sahn SA. Clinical features and outcome in patients with acute asthma presenting with hypercapnia. *Am Rev Respir Dis.* 1988;138:535-9.

60. Lougheed MD, Fisher T, O'Donnell DE. Dynamic hyperinflation during broncho constriction in asthma: implications for symptom perception. *Chest.* 2006;130:1072-81.

61. Reddy VG. Auto-PEEP: how to detect and how to prevent—a review. *Middle East J Anesthesiol.* 2005;18:293-312.

62. Tuxen DV. Permissive hypercapnic ventilation. *Am J Respir Crit Care Med.* 1994;150:870-4.

63. Papiris S, et al. Clinical review: severe asthma. *Crit Care.* 2002;6:30-44.

64. Manser R, Reid D, Abramson M. Corticosteroids for acute severe asthma in hospitalised patients. *Cochrane Database Syst Rev.* 2001;(1):CD001740.

65. Dhand R, Tobin MJ. Inhaled bronchodilator therapy in mechanically ventilated patients. *Am J Respir Crit Care Med.* 1997;156:3-10.

66. Maslow AD, et al. Inhaled albuterol, but not intravenous lidocaine, protects against intubation-induced bronchoconstriction in asthma. *Anesthesiology.* 2000;93:1198-204.

67. Behbehani NA, et al. Myopathy following mechanical ventilation for acute severe asthma: the role of muscle relaxants and corticosteroids. *Chest.* 1999;115:1627-31.

Pulmonary Exacerbations in Cystic Fibrosis

Patrick A Flume

INTRODUCTION

Cystic fibrosis (CF) is a genetic disease with multiple clinical manifestations including pancreatic insufficiency with malnutrition and chronic sinusitis, but it is the bronchiectasis and chronic airways infection that is the cause of the greatest morbidity and the shortening of life.[1] CF lung disease begins early in life with impaired mucociliary clearance and consequent chronic infection of the airways.[2] An exaggerated inflammatory response contributes to persistent injury to the airways.[3] The patient has daily symptoms of chronic airways infection, but there are also episodes of acute worsening of respiratory symptoms, often referred to as "pulmonary exacerbations". The clinical features of an exacerbation may include increased cough, increased sputum production, shortness of breath, chest pain, loss of appetite, loss of weight, and lung function decline.[4] Pulmonary exacerbations have a varying severity and often result in absence from work or school and there is an adverse impact on patient's quality of life.[5] Many result in hospitalization and thus have a major impact on the overall cost of care.[6] They are also associated with a further loss of lung function that is not fully recovered[7] and with earlier mortality.[8]

Pulmonary exacerbations are a common event. In 2008, there were 19,214 events, accounting for approximately 30% of clinical evaluations in that year.[1] These events are more common in patients with more advanced lung disease; the patients tend to be older and have a lower lung function (forced expiratory volume in 1 second (FEV_1) % predicted).[4] As it is such a common event, we have considerable experience with the diagnosis and management of CF pulmonary exacerbations. Yet, as was seen in the recent Cystic Fibrosis Foundation (CFF) Pulmonary Guidelines Committee recommendations on treatment of pulmonary exacerbations, there is a lack of sufficient information to define best practices.[9] What follows is a summary of what we know about the pathophysiology and treatment of CF pulmonary exacerbations.

PATHOGENESIS OF CF AIRWAYS DISEASE

An understanding of the CF pulmonary exacerbation requires knowledge of the underlying disease process. The pathogenesis of lung disease begins with gene mutations of the cystic fibrosis transmembrane conductance regulator (CFTR). This protein normally resides in the apical surface of the epithelial cell, but the mutations that cause CF result either in a reduction or abnormal function of CFTR such that overall CFTR activity is markedly reduced.[10] CFTR has been proposed to have several functions, but its role as an ion channel is a major contributor to the maintenance of the airway surface liquid and reduced CFTR activity results in a shallow airway surface liquid, preventing the cilia from standing erect and beating appropriately.[11] From the very beginning of life, patients with CF suffer from impaired mucociliary clearance.

For reasons that are not entirely clear, the reduction in CFTR activity and impaired mucociliary clearance allow for the establishment of chronic airways infection. Microaspiration allows entry of bacteria into the lower airways and they are not rapidly cleared by host defenses; therefore, these opportunists expand in numbers to create infection.[12] *Pseudomonas aeruginosa* is the most common bacterium isolated from the CF airways, but other Gram-negative bacteria, including *Achromobacter*, *Stenotrophomonas* and *Burkholderia*, can produce clinically significant chronic lung infections.[13] *Haemophilus influenzae* is often identified early in the course of chronic airway infection in CF. *Staphylococcus aureus* is the most commonly isolated Gram-positive species, and there is an increasing prevalence of methicillin-resistant *S. aureus* (MRSA) in the CF community.[13] Standard methods of bacterial culture typically reveal 1–3 pathogens, but molecular techniques of bacterial detection suggest that many more opportunistic bacterial species also may be present in chronic airway infections.[14]

Although CF clinicians have adopted a strategy of aggressive antibiotic use for first infection[15] in the hopes of eradicating bacteria[16] and delaying the time to development of chronic infection,[17] the latter is an inevitable result. Pulmonary infection is considered to be chronic when bacteria are consistently cultured from the airways over time,[18] often despite administration of antibiotics predicted to eradicate the organism based on *in vitro* susceptibility tests. The persistence of bacterial populations in the CF airways is no longer described as colonization because of the associated inflammatory response. However, the chronic bacterial infection of CF differs from acute lung infections in that the pathogens typically reside within the airways and rarely lead to invasive bacteremia; they are not generally associated with symptoms of acute infection[19] and the failure to eradicate these organisms is not directly associated with mortality.[20]

The host response is typically exuberant with much greater numbers of neutrophils than would be expected for a non-CF pulmonary infection.[21] The exaggerated inflammatory response further obstructs the airways with bacteria and cellular debris from the lysis of the large numbers of neutrophils.[3,22-24] The rapid degradation of these cells and release of their intracellular contents, including neutrophil-derived deoxyribonucleic acid (DNA) and filamentous actin (F-actin), further increase the viscosity and adhesivity of the airway secretions.[25,26] The secretions present in the CF airways, therefore, contain pathogenic bacteria and inflammatory cytokines that perpetuate the injury to the airways by recruiting new inflammatory cells.

A growing body of evidence suggests that lung damage resulting from chronic infection is mediated more through the host inflammatory response to bacterial antigens than from the direct action of secreted bacterial toxins or other virulence factors.[27] Thus, the degree to which an infecting bacterial species is pathogenic is difficult to define; there is a possibility that a bacterial strain could be more pathogenic in one host than another.

Thus, the CF patient lives with chronically infected and inflamed airways producing large amounts of phlegm and resulting in daily cough productive of purulent sputum. There are a number of medications available to treat CF airways disease with the intent to relieve the daily symptoms and to slow down the progression of disease.[28] Recommended medications address the disease process of obstruction (dornase alfa, hypertonic saline, and bronchodilators), infection (aerosolized antibiotics), and inflammation (ibuprofen, macrolides). The demonstrated benefit of these medications is in their improvement in lung function, slowing of the rate of decline of lung function (i.e., ibuprofen) and reducing the frequency of pulmonary exacerbations.

WHAT IS AN EXACERBATION?

The natural history of CF airways disease is one of the progressive losses of lung function with episodes of acute worsening of symptoms or pulmonary exacerbations. A pulmonary exacerbation is best described as an acute worsening of symptoms, typically an increase in cough and sputum production, but there are many other clinical features of exacerbations that have been described in table 3-1. All of these clinical manifestations are what might be predicted if there were worsening infection and inflammation with both local (e.g., cough and sputum) and systemic (e.g., fever and anorexia) effects. Existing definitions have been based upon empiric observations, but there is no accepted standard definition, although some definitions have been developed for the purpose of clinical trials.[29-32]

There is an obvious agreement on many aspects of a pulmonary exacerbation, but there are also striking differences (Table 3-1). For example, the Fuchs criteria included sinus symptoms and although worsening sinus infection could result in worsening lower airways infection, the approach to treatment may differ considerably in the absence of respiratory symptoms. Likewise, the occurrence of a pneumothorax clearly represents a pulmonary event but does not necessarily represent a pulmonary exacerbation. Recent guidelines on the treatment of a CF-related pneumothorax[33] do

Table 3-1 Definitions of CF Pulmonary Exacerbations

Sign or symptom	Fuchs[29]	Ramsey[32]	CFF Guidelines[68]	Rosenfeld[34]	Kraynack[69]	Rabin[35]	Blumer[70]
Cough	X	X	X	X	X	X	X
Sputum	X	X	X	X	X	X	X
Hemoptysis	X				X	X	
Dyspnea	X				X		X
Exercise tolerance			X	X	X		X
Absenteeism		X	X	X	X		X
Fatigue, malaise	X				X		X
Fever	X	X	X		X		
Weight loss	X	X	X	X	X	X	X
Sinus pain	X	X					
Sinus discharge	X						
Chest exam	X		X	X	X	X	X
Tachypnea		X	X				X
Lung function	X	X	X	X	X	X	X
CXR	X		X		X		
SaO2			X		X		
Neutrophilia		X					
Criteria	4 of 12 plus antibiotics	2 of 5 plus 1 of 3	3 of 11	Score	Score	3 of 4	5 of 10

CFF, Cystic Fibrosis Foundation.

not offer the same recommendations as in the treatment guidelines for pulmonary exacerbations.[9]

Some clinical features of a pulmonary exacerbation may be excessively weighted, especially a change in lung function (i.e., decrease in FEV_1). The one attempt to determine a validated definition of a pulmonary exacerbation noted that a change in FEV_1 added little to the sensitivity of the score;[34] yet, it is apparent that decreasing lung function significantly influences clinical decisions to treat. In fact, it has been the clinician's decision to treat that has complicated our current definitions. An analysis of a CF registry used the decision to treat for determining the most common clinical features of a pulmonary exacerbation.[35] Those criteria were then applied to the same dataset to define pulmonary exacerbations, finding that physicians treated only a fraction of the patients who met the criteria. This problem is not unique to CF; there is a high variability in existing definitions for COPD exacerbations, where there are approximately half as many exacerbations when defined as decision to treat compared to patient symptoms.[36]

We would like for a validated definition to inform the patient, family, and clinician that an intervention is necessary. An accepted definition should also account for severity, as some exacerbations may lead to hospitalization while others may be treated in the outpatient setting.

CAUSES OF AN EXACERBATION

As the pulmonary exacerbation is often considered an acute event, there have been several proposed causes that involve either a new infection, or a change in the chronic infection, or another acute injury to the airways. A new infection, either viral or bacterial, may incite an increase in inflammation.[37] Viral infection has been implicated, especially in younger patients with serologic testing, typically used to associate viruses with the event.[38-40] Bacteria are frequently introduced to the lower airways by aspiration and some may establish a local infection.[13] Some have proposed that a new organism is not required but that the bacteria chronically present in the airways undergo a change, altering their virulence or numbers.[41] Noninfectious injury to the airways may also incite an increased inflammatory response. Aspiration, possibly associated with gastroesophageal reflux disease, may cause local injury, even in the absence of any change in chronic infection.[42] Environmental pollution has been shown to have an association with increased frequency of exacerbations.[43] Although an exacerbation is described as an acute event, it is also possible that an exacerbation is the result of progressive chronic disease. In this hypothesis, the sequelae of the disease have exceeded a symptomatic threshold whereby now the patient seeks evaluation. In such cases, the signs and symptoms may be resolved simply by performance of usual chronic therapies.

TREATMENT OF AN EXACERBATION

There are recently published guidelines on the treatment of acute pulmonary exacerbations based upon a systematic review of the literature and including a variety of commonly used therapies[9] (Table 3-2). It is unlikely that the clinician will be able to determine a specific cause of a pulmonary exacerbation that would guide specific therapy for its resolution. Therefore, the treatment is typically based upon the supposition that there is a new infection, a change in the existing infection, and there is a progression of the underlying disease process. In keeping with the latter, the CF Pulmonary Guidelines Committee recommended that chronic therapies, including airway clearance therapies and medications, should be used in the treatment of an acute exacerbation. The Committee recommended an increased intensity of airway clearance therapies, either by an increased frequency or duration. The medications recommended for chronic use include dornase alfa, inhaled antibiotics, bronchodilators, oral macrolides, and oral ibuprofen.[28] In many cases, this aspect of treatment is most critical to the improvement in a patient's health and sense of well-being, as well as return lung function to its previous baseline.

Site of Treatment

Once the clinician has determined the need for an intervention, the next decision is where that treatment will take place. Since antibiotics are frequently a component of treatment (see below), the antibiotic choices often play a considerable role in deciding where treatment will occur. Oral and inhaled antibiotics are easily administered at home, and intravenous antibiotics can often be used in the home safely as well. There is one small randomized trial[44] and several observational studies[45-49] that have compared home and hospital antibiotic therapies. Lung function improves when treated in either site, and although there was no difference between sites in the controlled trial, the observational studies tended to favor the hospital setting. As for quality of life, hospital therapy tends to be more disruptive to family life than home therapy, but is less fatiguing.

The CF Pulmonary Guidelines recommended that home therapy could be appropriate, assuming all aspects of treatment are equivalent.[9] Some patients cannot be treated with home intravenous antibiotics because either they are too ill or they lack the financial (e.g., insurance) and ancillary (e.g., family) resources to guarantee success. The dosing regimens may be exhausting (e.g., four times daily), and fatigue or sleep deprivation may hinder performance of the other components of treatment. This is a critical aspect of the decision regarding the site of treatment; the treatment of an exacerbation involves more than just prescribing antibiotics. Many patients will be better served to be admitted to the hospital to focus on treatment components, such as airway clearance, that are critical to both short- and long-term treatment goals.

Table 3-2	Guidelines for Therapies Commonly Used to Treat CF Pulmonary Exacerbations	
	Recommendations	*Rating*
	The Cystic Fibrosis Foundation (CFF) recommends against the delivery of intravenous antibiotics in a nonhospital setting unless resources and support equivalent to the hospital setting can be assured for the treatment of an acute exacerbation of pulmonary disease.	I
	The CFF concludes that there is insufficient evidence to recommend for, or against continued use of inhaled antibiotics in patients treated with the same antibiotics intravenously for the treatment of an acute exacerbation of pulmonary disease.	I
	The CFF recommends continuing chronic therapies for maintenance of lung health during treatment of an acute exacerbation of pulmonary disease.	B
	The CFF recommends that airway clearance therapy be increased as part of the treatment of an acute exacerbation of pulmonary disease.	B
	The CFF concludes that there is insufficient evidence to recommend the use of a single antibiotic as being equivalent to the use of more than one antibiotic class for treatment of *Pseudomonas* infection during an acute exacerbation of pulmonary disease.	I
	The CFF recommends that once daily dosing of aminoglycosides is preferable to three-times daily dosing for treatment of an acute exacerbation of pulmonary disease.	C
	The CFF concludes that there is insufficient evidence to recommend the continuous infusion of beta-lactam antibiotics for the treatment of an acute exacerbation of pulmonary disease.	I
	The CFF concludes that there is insufficient evidence to recommend an optimal duration of antibiotic treatment of an acute exacerbation of pulmonary disease.	I
	The CFF recommends against the use of synergy testing as part of the routine evaluation of the patient with an acute exacerbation of pulmonary disease and multidrug-resistant bacteria.	D
	The CFF concludes that there is insufficient evidence to recommend the routine use of corticosteroids in the treatment of an acute exacerbation of pulmonary disease.	I

Ratings of recommendations are adapted from a published US Preventive Services Task Force Recommendation Statement.[50] The ratings are as follows:

A—High certainty that the net benefit is substantial.

B—High certainty that the net benefit is moderate or there is moderate certainty that the net benefit is moderate to substantial.

C—There may be considerations that support providing the service to an individual patient. There is moderate or high certainty that the net benefit is small.

D—There is moderate or high certainty that the service has no net benefit or that the harm outweighs the benefits.

I—Evidence is lacking, of poor quality, or conflicting, and the balance of benefits and harms cannot be determined.

Adapted from Cystic Fibrosis Foundation. Treatment of pulmonary exacerbation of cystic fibrosis. In: *Clinical Practice Guidelines for Cystic Fibrosis.* MD, USA: Bethesda. 1997.

Antibiotics

Antibiotics are commonly used to treat exacerbations, based upon the premise that worsening bacterial infection is either the cause or a complicating factor of an exacerbation. The antibiotics selected may be oral, inhaled, or intravenous and are typically selected based upon the knowledge of patient's previous sputum cultures. As noted in the section on the microbiology of the CF airways, the chronic infection typically includes multiple bacteria, only a few of which have been identified by standard culture testing. Also, there may be multiple strains of the same species, especially *P. aeruginosa*, with susceptibility test results that confound a selection of antibiotics which treat all bacterial organisms present in the culture. To complicate matters, there is often discordance between the results of microbiology susceptibility testing and the clinical outcomes of the patients treated with antibiotics. More specifically, it is not uncommon for patients to improve clinically with antibiotics even though culture data would suggest otherwise. As such, a common approach for the selection of antibiotics is to choose those which have been previously used successfully. When the patient does not improve satisfactorily, more recent culture data may be used to guide antibiotic changes.

Combinations of antibiotics are frequently used to treat CF pulmonary exacerbations. Some recommendations suggest that combinations of antibiotics are required to treat *Pseudomonas* infections offering reasons such as broader coverage in the event of antibiotic resistance, prevention of selection of resistant bacteria, and provision of synergistic antibacterial activity.[51-56] The first to these kinds is the premise behind empiric treatment of pneumonia in the intensive care unit; inadequate treatment of a resistant pathogen in an acute infection often results in a dire outcome.[57,58] However, as noted above, CF patients with a pulmonary xacerbation often improve even when the apparent pathogens are resistant to the antibiotics. Finally, antibiotic synergy has not been demonstrated to be clinically relevant in the treatment of CF pulmonary exacerbations,[59] and the guidelines do not recommend the routine use of synergy testing to guide therapy.[9] Although there is a paucity of data to support the need for combination of antibiotics to treat *Pseudomonas*, the CF Pulmonary Guidelines noted that there are no studies which have demonstrated that one antibiotic is equivalent to two. Although it may not be necessary to treat *Pseudomonas* infection alone with combination antibiotics, it may be shown that patients still do better with the combination of antibiotics because of the complexity of their chronic infection.

Recommendations for dosing of antibiotics are provided in table 3-3. The CF Pulmonary Guidelines recommended that once daily aminoglycosides was preferable to the traditional three times daily dosing.[9] There is a trend towards the use of extended infusion of beta-lactam antibiotics to take advantage of their pharmacodynamic properties,[60] but in the CF literature there was insufficient

Table 3-3	Antibiotic Dosing Recommendations for CF Pulmonary Exacerbations				
Drugs	Pathogens*	Oral dosing	IV dosing	IV drug monitoring	Inhaled**
Aminoglycosides					
Tobramycin	PA, HI		10 mg/kg/d divided every 12 h every 24 h	Peak 10–16 μg/mL Trough < 0.5 μg mL Peak 25–35 μg/mL Trough < 0.5 μg/mL	TIS 300 mg BID
Amikacin	PA, HI		30 mg/kg/d divided every 12 h every 24 h	Peak 15–20 μg/mL Trough < 5 μg/mL Peak 30–45 μg/mL Trough < 5 μg/mL	250–500 mg BID (off label use of IV formulation)
Penicillins					
Amoxicillin	MSSA	500 mg TID			
Piperacillin-tazobactam	PA, MSSA		4.5 g every 6 h		
Ticarcillin-clavulanate	PA, MSSA, SM		3.1 g every 4–6 h		
Cephalosporins					
Ceftazidime	PA, MSSA, HI		2 g every 8 h		250–500 mg BID (off label use of IV formulation)
Cefepime	PA, MSSA, HI		2 g every 8 h		

Continued

Continued

Drugs	Pathogens*	Oral dosing	IV dosing	IV drug monitoring	Inhaled**
Carbapenems					
Imipenem-cilastatin	PA, MSSA, HI		500 mg every 6 h		
Meropenem	PA, MSSA, HI		1–2 g every 8 h		
Doripenem	PA, MSSA, HI		500 mg every 8 h		
Monobactams					
Aztreonam	PA, MSSA, HI		2 g every 8 h		Aztreonam inhalation solution 75 mg TID
Fluoroquinolones					
Ciprofloxacin	PA, MSSA, HI	500–750 mg BID-TID	400 mg TID		
Levofloxacin	PA, MSSA, HI, SM	750–1000 mg BID	750 mg every 12–24 h		
Moxifloxacin	PA, MSSA, HI, SM	400 mg BID	400 mg daily		
Tetracyclines					
Tigecycline	MSSA, MRSA		100 mg × 1, then 50 mg every 12 h		
Doxycycline	MSSA, MRSA, SM	100 mg BID	100 mg BID		
Minocycline	MSSA, MRSA, HI	200 mg then 100 mg BID			
Others					
Vancomycin	MSSA, MRSA		15 mg/kg/d every 8–24 h	Trough 15–20 µg/mL	250–500 mg BID (off label use of IV formulation)

Continued

Continued

Drugs	Pathogens*	Oral dosing	IV dosing	IV drug monitoring	Inhaled**
Linezolid	MSSA, MRSA	600 mg BID	600 mg BID		
Trimethoprim-Sulfamethoxazole	MSSA, MRSA, SM	15–20 mg/kg/d trimethoprim divided every 6 h	15–20 mg/kg/d trimethoprim divided every 6 h		
Colistin	PA		2 mg/kg every 12 h		75 mg BID (off label use of IV formulation)
Chloramphenicol	HI, BC, SM	50–100 mg/kg/d divided every 6 h	50–100 mg/kg/d divided every 6 h	Maximum 4–8 g/day	

*The drugs generally have activity against these pathogens, but some organisms may be resistant.
**If drug trade name is provided then there is an FDA-approved product; all other dosing is off label use of intravenous formulations. CFF Pulmonary Guidelines recommend the use of TIS for patients who have *P. aeruginosa*,[9] but there is insufficient information to make a recommendation about such off-label use of medications. Inhaled aztreonam was approved by the FDA after publication of the Cystic Fibrosis Foundation (CFF) Pulmonary Guidelines on chronic medications and so did not have sufficient information for a recommendation at that time.

PA, *Pseudomonas aeruginosa*; MSSA, methicillin-sensitive *Staphylococcus aureus*; MRSA, methicillin-resistant *Staphylococcus aureus*; HI, *Haemophilus influenzae*; SM, *Stenotrophomonas maltophilia*; BC, *Burkholderia cepacia*; TIS, tobramycin inhalation solution.

CFF Pulmonary Guidelines have suggested that once daily dosing is as effective as three times daily dosing.

evidence to recommend continuous infusion of beta-lactam antibiotics. Intravenous dosing has been considered the gold standard of treatment and is typically used for more severe exacerbations. However, the bioavailability of most of the oral antibiotics has been demonstrated to be similar in CF patients to the general population and could be used when appropriate.[61] Aerosol delivery of antibiotics results in high concentrations of drugs in the airways, possibly at the site of infection, but there are no studies that have compared aerosol to intravenous treatment for exacerbations.

There are no studies that have investigated the optimal duration of antibiotic therapy. The median duration of intravenous antibiotics is 14–16 days,[1] but there is a considerable variation in practice.[9]

Corticosteroids

Corticosteroids are frequently used to treat exacerbations of other airways diseases (e.g., asthma, COPD) to acutely reduce inflammation. There is insufficient evidence at this time to know whether systemic corticosteroids are effective in CF pulmonary exacerbations.[9] Some patients with CF also have asthma or allergic bronchopulmonary aspergillosis (ABPA) (See below) and these patients may benefit from a burst of systemic corticosteroids.

COMPLICATIONS

There are other common pulmonary complications that are related to pulmonary exacerbations and warrant further discussion. Allergic bronchopulmonary aspergillosis (ABPA) occurs in a minority (8–10%) of CF patients[62] but an exacerbation in these patients could be due to the causes discussed earlier or be a manifestation of their allergic asthma. Pneumothorax and massive hemoptysis occur in less than 5% of patients and may not be a part of pulmonary exacerbation, but they typically results in hospitalization. They occur more commonly in patients with more advanced pulmonary disease. Respiratory failure is another manifestation of advanced lung disease and could be an aspect of a pulmonary exacerbation.

Allergic Bronchopulmonary Aspergillosis (ABPA)

ABPA is asthma that is the result of an allergy to a common fungus, *Aspergillus fumigatus*. It is a common disease that is found with greater frequency in patients with CF than in the general population.[62] The diagnosis is made principally by an elevated immunoglobulin E (IgE) level, antibodies to *Aspergillus* and an immediate histamine reaction to skin testing with *Aspergillus* antigen. Other clinical features of ABPA are common to CF (e.g., bronchiectasis, sputum production), and so may not be useful in the diagnosis in CF patients. There are guidelines on the diagnosis and management of ABPA in CF,[62] and so will not be discussed here further. The CFF Pulmonary Guidelines on Chronic Medications recommended against the routine use of inhaled and systemic steroids with the exclusion of patients who have asthma or ABPA.[28] Likewise, the CFF Guidelines on treatment of pulmonary exacerbations found insufficient information to make a recommendation about the use of steroids, but steroid therapy is commonly used to treat ABPA exacerbations,[62] and so they could be useful in CF pulmonary exacerbations in patients who also have ABPA. For such patients, it is often difficult to know whether it is the ABPA or other etiology of the exacerbation, but it may prove useful to measure an IgE level at the time of evaluation.

Pneumothorax

Pneumothorax occurs most commonly in patients who are older and have more advanced obstructive airways disease.[63] The average annual incidence of pneumothorax is 0.64% or 1 in 167 patients per year, and approximately 3.4% of individuals with CF will experience a pneumothorax during their lifetime.[63] It is not typically considered to be a manifestation of a pulmonary exacerbation, but frequently results in admission to the hospital. There are no prospective studies on proper management of a pneumothorax in CF patients, but there are consensus guidelines developed using unbiased assessment of expert opinion.[33]

It is beyond the scope of this monograph to review all of the recommendations, but there are few that are relevant to pulmonary exacerbations. The patient with a large pneumothorax should always be admitted to the hospital; whereas, the patient with a small pneumothorax, who is otherwise clinically stable, may be closely observed in the outpatient setting. The patient with a large pneumothorax should have a chest tube placed. On the other hand, the patient with a small pneumothorax should have a chest tube placed, only if there is clinical instability. Some panelists did not rate this statement higher, as there was a doubt that the small pneumothorax would be the cause of clinical instability and that treatment of a pulmonary exacerbation[9] would be more appropriate. Although some panelists suggested pneumothorax as a manifestation of a pulmonary exacerbation, others required additional evidence of a pulmonary exacerbation before treating the patient with antibiotics. Some airway clearance therapies, specifically positive expiratory pressure and intrapulmonary percussive ventilation, should not be used in patients with pneumothorax. The patient with pneumothorax should not stop aerosol therapies, even though some can be irritating to the airways and induce cough and bronchospasm in some patients.[31] Although there were higher ratings for hypertonic saline, they were not so high as to change the recommendation.

Hemoptysis

Hemoptysis is common in patients with CF, but the bleeding is most commonly scant to moderate. However, massive and life-threatening bleeding can occur.

Approximately 4.1% of all patients with CF will suffer massive hemoptysis during their lifetime, and the average annual incidence is 0.87% or 1 in 115 patients per year.[64] In many cases, bleeding of any amount is considered to be a manifestation of a pulmonary exacerbation and treatment will be the same. There are now consensus guidelines developed using unbiased assessment of expert opinion.[33]

It is beyond the scope of this chapter to review all of the recommendations, but there are some that are relevant to pulmonary exacerbations. First, the patient with at least mild hemoptysis (≥ 5 mL) should contact their healthcare provider as this amount suggests an acute problem and treatment may be warranted. Second, not all bleeding must be treated in the hospital, but the patient with massive hemoptysis should always be admitted to the hospital. As the hemoptysis may well be a manifestation of a pulmonary exacerbation,[65] the Committee recommended that the patient with at least mild (≥ 5 mL) hemoptysis should be treated with antibiotics. The Committee recommended that airway clearance therapies should be continued unless there is massive hemoptysis, when all forms of airway clearance should be stopped. This is not because it is believed that airway clearance therapies cause hemoptysis, but they may impair clot formation and adherence resulting in more bleeding. Similarly, aerosol medications are recommended to be continued in the treatment of pulmonary exacerbation and the CF guidelines on complications did not recommend stopping them for hemoptysis. However, in the setting of massive hemoptysis, the Committee felt that hypertonic saline should be discontinued, again not because it caused the bleeding but because it may be irritating to the airways and induce cough in some patients[31] and possibly aggravate the hemoptysis. Finally, bronchial artery embolization (BAE) is appropriate for some patients with massive hemoptysis, either because of clinical instability or because of persistent bleeding. The committee was unresolved about the need to perform chest tomography (CT) prior to BAE; however, they recommended that the patient with massive hemoptysis should not undergo bronchoscopy prior to BAE, as it offered a little benefit and would delay performance of the procedure.

Respiratory Failure

As stated earlier, the natural history of CF lung disease is a progression to eventual respiratory failure. There is no real difference in how to manage hypercapnic or hypoxic respiratory failure due to CF lung disease compared to any other advanced stage obstructive airways disease. Oxygen supplementation is provided using the same parameters as for any other lung disease. Hypercapnic respiratory failure can be managed with ventilatory support, but intubation and mechanical ventilation for CF patients with advanced stage lung disease has an extremely poor prognosis, and for many patients it is not an advisable treatment option unless they are listed for lung transplantation. Noninvasive ventilatory support using bi-level positive airway pressure (BiPAP) has been used with success as a palliative measure.[66]

CASE STUDY

A 22-year-old male with CF presents to clinic with complaints of an increase in cough and sputum production over the last week. The sputum has become darker in color, and there is a streaky hemoptysis associated with the cough. There is no fever or chest pain. He feels more fatigued but there is no shortness of breath. His appetite has diminished and he feels that he may have lost weight.

On examination he is afebrile, his weight is 73.2 kg, which is decreased from his baseline of 77.1 kg. Pulse oximetry reveals an arterial oxygen saturation of 97% on room air. His chest exam reveals crackles in both upper lung zones; those on the right are new since the last exam, but there is no wheeze. He has chronic clubbing to his fingers.

His current medications include dornase alfa nebulized daily, inhaled tobramycin twice daily, albuterol by metered dose inhaled twice daily, hypertonic saline nebulized twice daily, azithromycin orally daily, digestive enzymes and multivitamins. His usual form of airway clearance therapy is oscillatory positive expiratory pressure using an Acapella device, but he admits that he has not been consistent with its use. His current spirometry measures are reduced from his baseline measures (Figure 3-1). His current and previous chest radiographs are shown in figure 3-2; there are no new findings.

The clinician makes the diagnosis of an acute pulmonary exacerbation, and the decision is made to begin treatment in the hospital. Previously, he had been treated successfully with ceftazidime and tobramycin, and so these antibiotics are initiated. He is also started on his chronic therapies, but the inhaled tobramycin is

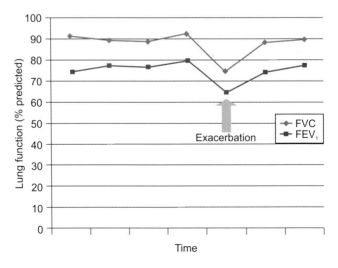

Figure 3-1 Findings on spirometry.

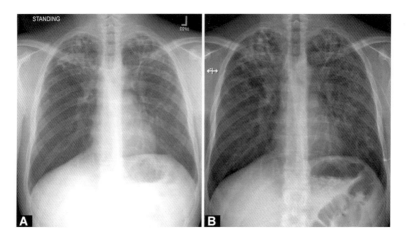

Figure 3-2 **A,** Baseline CXR performed when in stable condition. **B,** CXR performed at time of pulmonary exacerbation.

withheld. Respiratory therapist begins chest physiotherapy (CPT) and introduces him to high frequency chest compression.[67]

After 4 days of therapy the sputum culture, obtained at admission, has grown two strains of *Pseudomonas aeruginosa* both of which are resistant to ceftazidime and tobramycin, but are susceptible to ciprofloxacin and piperacillin-tazobactam. The patient feels considerably better with less fatigue, a greater appetite, and less cough and sputum production. The clinician decides to continue with the present therapy despite the culture results, and on the fifth day, the patient is discharged from the hospital to complete a total of 14 days of intravenous antibiotics. At the completion of this therapy, the patient returns to clinic for removal of the PICC line and spirometry has returned to the previous baseline (Figure 3-1).

CONCLUSION

The CF pulmonary exacerbation is a common event in the natural history of CF lung disease. Clinicians generally feel comfortable with the identification and management of exacerbation. Yet, one of the critical findings of the systematic review for the CF pulmonary guidelines for the treatment of exacerbations was the paucity of evidence to support commonly used therapies. We recognized that treatment choices are highly variable, and there is no consensus as to which treatment is best. However, it is likely that some approaches to treatment are better than others and if we want to optimize treatment and improve outcomes, we will need to better describe and define the pulmonary exacerbation.

Once we have a validated definition, we can begin to address basic treatment questions that remain unanswered. We can better identify exacerbations so that we will know when we must treat them; this could be used as part of a center's quality initiative to improve the overall health of their patients. This could also become an important clinical endpoint to be used in clinical trials, evaluating chronic therapies to maintain lung health. Presumably, the definition would be responsive to therapy so we could assess acute therapies of exacerbations. We can then learn how to treat them best such as determining the optimal antibiotic duration and whether to use single or combination antibiotics.

REFERENCES

1. Cystic Fibrosis Foundation. Cystic Fibrosis Foundation Patient Registry 2008 Annual Data Report to the Center Directors. MD, USA: Bethesda. 2009.
2. Robinson M, Bye PT. Mucociliary clearance in cystic fibrosis. *Pediatr Pulmonol.* 2002; 33:293-306.
3. Konstan MW, Hilliard KA, Norvell TM, et al. Bronchoalveolar lavage findings in cystic fibrosis patients with stable, clinically mild lung disease suggest ongoing infection and inflammation. *Am J Respir Crit Care Med.* 1994;150:448-54.
4. Goss CH, Burns JL. Exacerbations in cystic fibrosis. 1: Epidemiology and pathogenesis. *Thorax.* 2007;62:360-7.
5. Britto MT, Kotagal UR, Hornung RW, et al. Impact of recent pulmonary exacerbations on quality of life in patients with cystic fibrosis. *Chest.* 2002;121:64-72.
6. Lieu TA, Ray GT, Farmer G, et al. The cost of medical care for patients with cystic fibrosis in a health maintenance organization. *Pediatrics.* 1999;103:e72.
7. Sanders DB, Hoffman LR, Emerson J, et al. Return of FEV1 after pulmonary exacerbation in children with cystic fibrosis. *Pediatr Pulmonol.* 2010;45:127-34.
8. Mayer-Hamblett N, Rosenfeld M, Emerson J, et al. Developing cystic fibrosis lung transplant referral criteria using predictors of 2-year mortality. *Am J Respir Crit Care Med.* 2002;166:1550-5.
9. Flume PA, Mogayzel PJ, Robinson KA, et al. Cystic Fibrosis Pulmonary Guidelines: treatment of pulmonary exacerbations. *Am J Respir Crit Care Med.* 2009;180:802-8.
10. Rowntree RK, Harris A. The phenotypic consequences of CFTR mutations. *Ann Hum Genet.* 2003;67:471-85.
11. Boucher RC. Evidence for airway surface dehydration as the initiating event in CF airway disease. *J Int Med.* 2007;261:5-16.
12. Lipuma JJ, VanDevanter DR. Unique aspects of chronic airways infections. *Comment Chron Airways Infect.* 2007;1:2-6.
13. Lipuma JJ. The changing microbial epidemiology in cystic fibrosis. *Clin Microbiol Rev.* 2010;23:299-323.
14. Rogers GB, Carroll MP, Serisier DJ, et al. Characterization of bacterial community diversity in cystic fibrosis lung infections by use of 16s ribosomal DNA terminal restriction fragment length polymorphism profiling. *J Clin Microbiol.* 2004;42:5176-83.
15. Cystic Fibrosis Foundation, Borowitz D, Robinson KA, et al. Cystic Fibrosis Foundation evidence-based guidelines for management of infants with cystic fibrosis. *J Pediatr.* 2009;155:S73-93.
16. Ratjen F, Munck A, Kho P, et al. Treatment of early *Pseudomonas aeruginosa* infection in patients with cystic fibrosis: the ELITE trial. *Thorax.* 2010;65:286-91.

17. Frederiksen B, Koch C, Hoiby N. Changing epidemiology of *Pseudomonas aeruginosa* infection in Danish cystic fibrosis patients (1974-1995). *Pediatr Pulmonol.* 1999;28: 159-66.

18. Lee TW, Brownlee KG, Conway SP, et al. Evaluation of a new definition for chronic *Pseudomonas aeruginosa* infection in cystic fibrosis patients. *J Cyst Fibr.* 2003;2:29-34.

19. Hoiby N, Krogh Johansen H, Moser C, et al. *Pseudomonas aeruginosa* and the *in vitro* and *in vivo* biofilm mode of growth. *Microbes Infect.* 2001;3:23-35.

20. Van Devanter DR. The value of *in vitro* susceptibility testing in guiding antibiotic choices for treatment of acute exacerbation. *Comment Chron Airways Infect.* 2007;1:8-13.

21. Muhlebach MS, Stewart PW, Leigh MW, et al. Quantitation of inflammatory responses to bacteria in young cystic fibrosis and control patients. *Am J Respir Crit Care Med.* 1999;160:186-91.

22. Birrer P, McElvaney NG, Rudeberg A, et al. Protease-antiprotease imbalance in the lungs of children with cystic fibrosis. *Am J Respir Crit Care Med.* 1994;150:207-13.

23. Bonfield TL, Konstan MW, Burfeind P, et al. Normal bronchial epithelial cells constitutively produce the anti-inflammatory cytokine interleukin-10, which is downregulated in cystic fibrosis. *Am J Respir Cell Mol Biol.* 1995;13:257-61.

24. Bonfield TL, Panuska JR, Konstan MW, et al. Inflammatory cytokines in cystic fibrosis lungs. *Am J Respir Crit Care Med.* 1995;152:2111-8.

25. Chernick WS, Barbero GJ. Composition of tracheobronchial secretions in cystic fibrosis of the pancreas and bronchiectasis. *Pediatrics.* 1959;24:739-45.

26. Vasconcellos CA, Allen PG, Wohl ME, et al. Reduction in viscosity of cystic fibrosis sputum in vitro by gelsolin. Science 1994;263:969-71.

27. Chmiel JF, Konstan MW. Inflammation and anti-inflammatory therapies for cystic fibrosis. *Clin Chest Med.* 2007;28:331-46.

28. Flume PA, O'Sullivan BP, Robinson KA, et al. Cystic Fibrosis Pulmonary Guidelines: chronic medications for maintenance of lung health. *Am J Respir Crit Care Med.* 2007; 176:957-69.

29. Fuchs HJ, Borowitz DS, Christiansen DH, et al. Effect of aerosolized recombinant human DNase on exacerbations of respiratory symptoms and on pulmonary function in patients with cystic fibrosis. The Pulmozyme Study Group. *N Engl J Med.* 1994;331:637-42.

30. Equi A, Balfour-Lynn IM, Bush A, et al. Long term azithromycin in children with cystic fibrosis: a randomised, placebo-controlled crossover trial. *Lancet.* 2002;360:978-84.

31. Elkins MR, Bye PT. Inhaled hypertonic saline as a therapy for cystic fibrosis. *Curr Opin Pulm Med.* 2006;12:445-52.

32. Ramsey BW, Astley SJ, Aitken ML, et al. Efficacy and safety of short-term administration of aerosolized recombinant human deoxyribonuclease in patients with cystic fibrosis. *Am Rev Respir Dis.* 1993;148:145-51.

33. Flume PA, Mogayzel PJ, Robinson KA, et al. Cystic Fibrosis Pulmonary Guidelines: pulmonary complications: hemoptysis and pneumothorax. *Am J Res Crit Care Med.* 2010;182:298-306.

34. Rosenfeld M, Emerson J, Williams-Warren J, et al. Defining a pulmonary exacerbation in cystic fibrosis. *J Pediatr.* 2001;139:359-65.

35. Rabin HR, Butler SM, Wohl ME, et al. Pulmonary exacerbations in cystic fibrosis. *Pediatr Pulmonol.* 2004;37:400-6.

36. Seemungal TA, Donaldson GC, Bhowmik A, et al. Time course and recovery of exacerbations in patients with chronic obstructive pulmonary disease. *Am J Respir Crit Care Med.* 2000;161:1608-13.

37. Aaron SD, Ramotar K, Ferris W, et al. Adult cystic fibrosis exacerbations and new strains of *Pseudomonas aeruginosa*. *Am J Respir Crit Care Med*. 2004;169:811-5.

38. Conway SP, Simmonds EJ, Littlewood JM. Acute severe deterioration in cystic fibrosis associated with influenza A virus infection. *Thorax*. 1992;47:112-4.

39. Ortiz JR, Neuzil KM, Victor JC, et al. Influenza-associated cystic fibrosis pulmonary exacerbations. *Chest*. 2010;137:852-60.

40. Abman SH, Ogle JW, Butler-Simon N, et al. Role of respiratory syncytial virus in early hospitalizations for respiratory distress of young infants with cystic fibrosis. *J Pediatr*. 1988;113:826-30.

41. Van Devanter DR, Van Dalfsen JM. How much do *Pseudomonas* biofilms contribute to symptoms of pulmonary exacerbation in cystic fibrosis? *Pediatr Pulmonol*. 2005;39: 504-6.

42. Orenstein SR. Respiratory complications of reflux disease in infants. In: Stein MR (Ed): Gastroesophageal Reflux Disease and Airway Disease. New York: Marcel Dekker; 1999. pp 269-84.

43. Goss CH, Newsom SA, Schildcrout JS, et al. Effect of ambient air pollution on pulmonary exacerbations and lung function in cystic fibrosis. *Am J Respir Crit Care Med*. 2004;169: 816-21.

44. Wolter JM, Bowler SD, Nolan PJ, et al. Home intravenous therapy in cystic fibrosis: a prospective randomized trial examining clinical, quality of life and cost aspects. *Eur Respir J*. 1997;10:896-900.

45. Bosworth DG, Nielson DW. Effectiveness of home versus hospital care in the routine treatment of cystic fibrosis. *Pediatr Pulmonol*. 1997;24:42-7.

46. Bradley JM, Wallace ES, Elborn JS, et al. An audit of the effect of intravenous antibiotic treatment on spirometric measures of pulmonary function in cystic fibrosis. *Irish J Med Sci*. 1999;168:25-8.

47. Nazer D, Abdulhamid I, Thomas R, et al. Home versus hospital intravenous antibiotic therapy for acute pulmonary exacerbations in children with cystic fibrosis. *Pediatr Pulmonol*. 2006;41:744-9.

48. Thornton J, Elliott RA, Tully MP, et al. Clinical and economic choices in the treatment of respiratory infections in cystic fibrosis: comparing hospital and home care. *J Cyst Fibr*. 2005;4:239-47.

49. Yi MS, Tsevat J, Wilmott RW, et al. The impact of treatment of pulmonary exacerbations on the health-related quality of life of patients with cystic fibrosis: does hospitalization make a difference? *J Pediatr*. 2004;144:711-8.

50. Sawaya GF, Guirguis-Blake J, LeFevre M, et al. Update on the methods of the US Preventive Services Task Force: Estimating certainty and magnitude of net benefit. *Ann Int Med*. 2007;147:871-5.

51. American Thoracic Society; Infectious Diseases Society of America. Guidelines for the management of adults with hospital-acquired, ventilator-associated, and healthcare-associated pneumonia. *Am J Respir Crit Care Med*. 2005;171:388-416.

52. Doring G, Conway SP, Heijerman HG, et al. Antibiotic therapy against *Pseudomonas aeruginosa* in cystic fibrosis: a European consensus. *Eur Respir J*. 2000;16:749-67.

53. Watkins J, Francis J, Kuzemko JA. Does monotherapy of pulmonary infections in cystic fibrosis lead to early development of resistant strains of *Pseudomonas aeruginosa? Scand J Gastroenterol Suppl*. 1988;143:81-5.

54. Weiss K, Lapointe JR. Routine susceptibility testing of four antibiotic combinations for improvement of laboratory guide to therapy of cystic fibrosis infections caused by *Pseudomonas aeruginosa. Antimicrob Agents Chemother*. 1995;39:2411-4.

55. Saiman L, Mehar F, Niu WW, et al. Antibiotic susceptibility of multiply resistant *Pseudomonas aeruginosa* isolated from patients with cystic fibrosis, including candidates for transplantation. *Clin Infect Dis.* 1996;23:532-7.

56. Saiman L. Clinical utility of synergy testing for multidrug-resistant *Pseudomonas aeruginosa* isolated from patients with cystic fibrosis: the motion for. *Paediatr Respir Rev.* 2007;8:249-55.

57. Kollef MH, Ward S, Sherman G, et al. Inadequate treatment of nosocomial infections is associated with certain empiric antibiotic choices. *Crit Care Med.* 2000;28:3456-64.

58. Kollef MH, Morrow LE, Baughman RP, et al. Health care-associated pneumonia (HCAP): a critical appraisal to improve identification, management, and outcomes—proceedings of the HCAP Summit. *Clin Infect Dis.* 2008;46:s296-334; quiz 335-8.

59. Aaron SD, Vandemheen KL, Ferris W, et al. Combination antibiotic susceptibility testing to treat exacerbations of cystic fibrosis associated with multiresistant bacteria: a randomised, double-blind, controlled clinical trial. *Lancet.* 2005;366:463-71.

60. McKinnon PS, Davis SL. Pharmacokinetic and pharmacodynamic issues in the treatment of bacterial infectious diseases. *Eur J Clin Microbiol Infect Dis.* 2004;23:271-88.

61. Bosso JA, Flume PA, Gray SL. Linezolid pharmacokinetics in adult patients with cystic fibrosis. *Antimicrob Agents Chemother.* 2004;48:281-4.

62. Stevens DA, Moss RB, Kurup VP, et al. Allergic bronchopulmonary aspergillosis in cystic fibrosis—state of the art: Cystic Fibrosis Foundation Consensus Conference. *Clin Infect Dis.* 2003;37:s225-64.

63. Flume PA, Strange C, Ye X, et al. Pneumothorax in cystic fibrosis. *Chest.* 2005;128: 720-8.

64. Flume PA, Yankaskas JR, Ebeling M, et al. Massive hemoptysis in cystic fibrosis. *Chest.* 2005;128:729-38.

65. Gibson RL, Burns JL, Ramsey BW. Pathophysiology and management of pulmonary infections in cystic fibrosis. *Am J Respir Crit Care Med.* 2003;168:918-51.

66. Moran F, Bradley JM, Piper AJ. Noninvasive ventilation for cystic fibrosis. [Update of *Cochrane Database Syst Rev.* 2007;(4):CD002769;PMID:17943773]. *Cochrane Database Syst Rev.* 2009;(1):CD002769.

67. Flume PA, Robinson KA, O'Sullivan BP, et al. Cystic fibrosis pulmonary guidelines: airway clearance therapies. *Respir Care.* 2009;54:522-37.

68. Cystic Fibrosis Foundation. Treatment of pulmonary exacerbation of cystic fibrosis. In: *Clinical Practice Guidelines for Cystic Fibrosis.* MD, USA: Bethesda. 1997.

69. Kraynack NC, McBride JT. Improving care at cystic fibrosis centers through quality improvement. *Semin Respir Crit Care Med.* 2009;30:547-58.

70. Blumer JL, Saiman L, Konstan MW, et al. The efficacy and safety of meropenem and tobramycin vs ceftazidime and tobramycin in the treatment of acute pulmonary exacerbations in patients with cystic fibrosis. *Chest.* 2005;128:2336-46.

Pulmonary Exacerbations in Bronchiectasis

Patrick A Flume

INTRODUCTION

Bronchiectasis is a structural disease of the airways, where there is a permanent dilatation of the bronchi.[1] The diagnosis is typically established by radiographic findings and can range from focal to diffuse and mild (Figure 4-1A) to severe (Figure 4-1B) involvement. There are numerous conditions that cause and are associated with bronchiectasis (Table 4-1), and therefore, there is a broad presentation of disease. Cystic fibrosis (CF) is one of the known diseases associated with bronchiectasis but the airways disease in these patients is different enough to be discussed separately (see Chapter 3 on CF), while all others are lumped into the broad category of non-CF bronchiectasis. Descriptive terms, such as cylindrical, varicose, saccular, or cystic bronchiectasis, are frequently used in the discussion of bronchiectasis, but generally these are not useful in determining the cause of bronchiectasis or treatment of disease. As radiographic scoring systems to define severity are improved, perhaps such descriptions may become more useful.

The prevalence of bronchiectasis is unknown, but there is a greater recognition of the condition with the advent of high-resolution chest tomography (HRCT)[2] and there is an increase in the prevalence of disease with age.[3] Patients tend to be older at

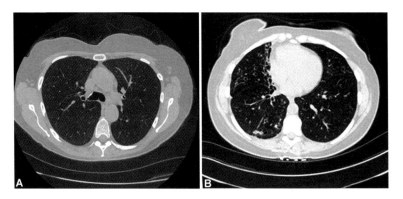

Figure 4-1 Bronchiectasis. **A,** Mild. **B,** Severe.

Table 4-1	Predisposing Factors and Associated Conditions with Bronchiectasis
Bronchial obstruction	**Immune-related infections**
Foreign body	Immunoglobulin deficiency
Bronchial stricture (e.g., compression by lymph nodes)	HIV/AIDS
	Post-transplant obliterative bronchiolitis
Endobronchial mass	
	Inhalation/aspiration
Bronchopulmonary infections	Aspiration with gastroesophageal reflux
Bacterial (e.g., pertussis, pneumonia)	
Mycobacterial (e.g., tuberculosis)	**Other associated conditions**
Viral (measles, influenza)	Allergic bronchopulmonary aspergillosis
	Rheumatoid arthritis
Congenital/hereditary conditions	Sjögren's syndrome
Cystic fibrosis	Inflammatory bowel disease
Primary ciliary dyskinesia	Relapsing polychondritis
Polycystic kidney disease	Yellow nail syndrome
Alfa-1-antitrypsin deficiency	

the time of diagnosis, although there are some conditions in which disease is found in the very young, such as CF.

The pathophysiology of bronchiectasis is discussed below, but it is generally associated with a persistent inflammatory state.[4] The disease is either caused by infection or, because of the structural changes, become vulnerable to chronic infection. Thus, the patient typically suffers from persistent cough and sputum production, and the sputum is often purulent. There is considerable morbidity associated with the disease, including dyspnea, chest pain and hemoptysis, and the patients are susceptible to acute exacerbations of disease, described as an acute worsening of symptoms that may result in admission to the hospital. What follows is a summary of what we know about the pathophysiology and treatment of non-CF pulmonary exacerbations.

PATHOGENESIS OF BRONCHIECTASIS

Bronchiectasis is a structural change of the bronchi and bronchioles, and is thought to be the result of remodeling in the setting of infection and inflammation.[4] A common pathway that is consistent with the pathogenesis of most-known associated diseases is shown in figure 4-2 with the theory that infection begets inflammation which causes injury to the airway; this further causes impaired mucociliary clearance, which, in turn, allows for persistence of infection. There is considerable inflammation in response to the chronic infection and the damage of the airways contributes further to the injury.

There are many conditions associated with the bronchiectasis (Table 4-1), and attempts to establish a causative diagnosis are important, as there may be specific

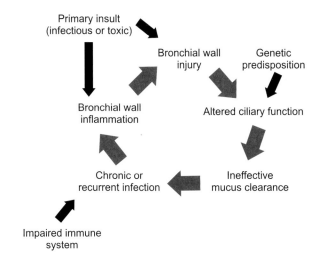

Figure 4-2 Common pathway for the pathogenesis of bronchiectasis.

therapies indicated for those patients. For example, allergic bronchopulmonary aspergillosis (ABPA) often responds to treatment with systemic corticosteroids.[5,6]

Focal bronchiectasis is the result of a discrete problem such as a previous infection or obstruction of the airway by either internal (e.g., foreign body[7]) or external (e.g., lymph nodes[8]) processes. Diffuse bronchiectasis may be associated with congenital disease or other systemic conditions. Ciliary dyskinesias are increasingly identified, and now there are identified associated genetic abnormalities.[9,10] Primary ciliary dyskinesia (PCD), an autosomal recessive disorder, is a condition of poorly functioning cilia that results in impaired mucociliary clearance and retention of secretions.[10,11] This is similar to CF in that there is an impaired mucociliary clearance, but, unlike CF, there is no disorder of the airway surface liquid. In classic PCD, a structural defect of the cilia can be seen, e.g., an absence of the dynein arms, but there is an increasing evidence of other functional abnormalities in the absence of a demonstrated structural defect.[12] Bronchiectasis has been demonstrated in patients with polycystic kidney disease;[13] and as this is a genetic disease associated with a sensory cilia abnormality, one could hypothesize that the bronchiectasis is also related to a ciliary defect.

Aspiration has been implicated as a cause of diffuse bronchiectasis, often associated with gastroesophageal reflux disease.[14-16] Immune deficiencies have been associated with bronchiectasis with a presumed mechanisms being an impaired response to injury or infection. Deficiencies of immunoglobulins IgG, IgM, and IgA have been associated with recurrent suppurative sinopulmonary infections and bronchiectasis.[17] Immunoglobulin replacement may reduce the frequency of infectious episodes.[18-20] The role of IgG subclass deficiency is controversial.[21-23] Rheumatologic conditions, most notably rheumatoid arthritis,[24,25] have been associated with bronchiectasis.[26]

Central bronchiectasis is one of the primary clinical features of the diagnosis of ABPA.[27,28] Other major diagnostic criteria include the presence of asthma, pulmonary infiltrates noted on chest radiograph, peripheral eosinophilia, an elevated total IgE (often markedly elevated), antibodies specific to *Aspergillus fumigatus*, and immediate cutaneous reactivity to *Aspergillus* species.[5,6] Other diagnostic elements commonly associated with ABPA include the production of plugs or sputum that is brown, sputum containing *A. fumigatus* either in culture or smear, and thickening of the airway walls suggesting bronchial inflammation, but these are considered as minor criteria of the diagnosis.[5,6] The disease is essentially an allergic asthma with a hypersensitivity to *Aspergillus* antigens. Corticosteroids are often effective in the treatment of disease and inhaled steroids may be sufficient to suppress inflammation.[5,6] Although this is not an actual fungal infection, antifungal therapy, such as voriconazole, may be effective in reducing the need for corticosteroids, presumably by reducing the burden of *Aspergillus* present in the airways.[5,6,29] There are recent data suggesting that omalizumab (anti-IgE) may also be effective therapy.[30]

Other infectious organisms have been often reported to be the cause of bronchiectasis with most recent interest in nontuberculous mycobacteria (NTM).[31,32] It is well known that severe pulmonary infection by *Mycobacterium tuberculosis* can result in permanent bronchiectasis[33] and so it is reasonable that other NTM might be considered as causes of bronchiectasis. An abnormal host defense may allow for the development of chronic NTM infection; genetic abnormalities have been described in families that have NTM infection,[34,35] suggesting some predisposition to such an infection. However, it may also be possible that the bronchiectasis precedes the NTM infection, and it is the abnormal airways that allows NTM to infect the airways as may occur in patients with CF.[36]

There are other examples of a genetic susceptibility for developing bronchiectasis. Because of the similarities between CF and non-CF bronchiectasis, an analysis of the CFTR gene was made in 50 adults with non-CF bronchiectasis.[37] Ten (20%) of these patients were ultimately diagnosed with CF and 8 (16%) subjects had an abnormal sweat chloride test of 40–60 mEq/dL, which is considered indeterminate for the diagnosis of CF. Fourteen of the remaining 32 patients had one identified CFTR mutation, a significantly higher carrier rate than seen in the general population. These findings suggest that altered CFTR function may be partially responsible for the development of bronchiectasis in these patients.

MICROBIOLOGY OF BRONCHIECTASIS

Bacteria are commonly present in the airways of patient with bronchiectasis. Microaspiration allows entry of bacteria into the lower airways and they are not rapidly cleared by host defenses, and therefore, these opportunists expand in numbers to create infection. The most frequently isolated bacteria are *Haemophilus influenzae* and *Pseudomonas aeruginosa*, but other Gram-negative bacteria, including *Achromobacter, Stenotrophomonas,* and *Burkholderia* can be found.[38] *Staphylococcus aureus* is the most commonly isolated Gram-positive species and there is an increasing prevalence of methicillin-resistant *S. aureus* (MRSA). The presence of *P. aeruginosa* is associated with increased sputum production, more extensive bronchiectasis visible on computed tomography (CT) of the chest,[39,40] more frequent exacerbations,[41] and reduced quality of life.[42-44]

Mycobacterial infection is also common in non-CF bronchiectasis,[45] whereas NTM affects approximately 13% of patients with CF;[36] the true prevalence for patients with non-CF bronchiectasis is not known, but reports range from 2 to 10%.[31,32] Most commonly, the organism is *Mycobacterium avium* complex (MAC) or *M. abscessus.*

Fungi, especially *Aspergillus fumigatus*, are also frequently cultured in non-CF bronchiectasis, but the clinical significance is often uncertain. For most of the fungi, a positive sputum culture is likely of no consequence and requires no specific treatment. However, for immunocompromised patients, a fungus is more likely to be clinically significant, especially if disease is suggested by nodular infiltrates on a CT of the chest.

MANAGEMENT OF CHRONIC BRONCHIECTASIS

A brief discussion of typical management of chronic bronchiectasis is relevant, as it has implications in the treatment of exacerbations. If there is a known cause of bronchiectasis (e.g., ABPA, immune globulin deficiency), appropriate therapy directed at that disease is indicated.[38] The daily treatment of non-CF bronchiectasis is similar in many ways to that of CF-related bronchiectasis; that is, clearance of airway secretions and treatment of the chronic infection and inflammation. Many of the therapies used to treat CF airways disease may be used in the management of non-CF bronchiectasis, but not all have the same beneficial results.

Aerosolized Antibiotics

Aerosolized antibiotics are commonly used to suppress chronic infection of the airways of the CF patient,[46] but they have not seen the same success in the non-CF bronchiectasis patient. Inhaled tobramycin is indicated in the treatment of CF patients with chronic airways infection with *P. aeruginosa*, but studies in non-CF bronchiectasis did not yield the same results.[47] There was a marked reduction in the density of *P. aeruginosa*, consistent with the antibacterial effect, but there was no change in forced expiratory volume in 1 second (FEV_1), as had been demonstrated in patients with CF. Aerosolized antibiotics may yet improve symptoms and quality of life in patients,[48] but the therapy has not been approved for use in patients with non-CF bronchiectasis.

Airway Clearance Therapies

Airway clearance therapies have long been a main component of CF airways treatment. The goal is to reduce the airways obstruction and decrease the overall burden of pathogens and concomitant inflammation. There is no consensus about the utility of daily airway clearance in non-CF bronchiectasis, although some patients certainly benefit from this practice.[49] Patients with non-CF bronchiectasis may not have the same degree of airways obstruction as in CF, but the principles are the same. The various methods for airways clearance include chest physiotherapy, active cycle breathing technique, autogenic drainage, and devices such as oscillating positive expiratory pressure (PEP) therapy (i.e., Flutter, Acapella), oscillating compression vest therapy, and intrapulmonary percussive ventilation. No single modality has been proven superior to the others, although patients typically express preference for methods they may use independently.

Medications that Alter Airways Secretions

Airway clearance can be augmented by agents that change the rheology of sputum, making it easier to expectorate, or by agents that enhance mucociliary clearance. A complete discussion of these agents is beyond the scope of this commentary, but dornase alfa and hypertonic saline are commonly used as such in patients with CF.[46] Dornase alfa has been studied extensively in patients with CF and has shown improved pulmonary function and a reduction in the number of acute exacerbations.[50] A clinical trial of dornase alfa in patients with non-CF bronchiectasis did not demonstrate the same benefits and actually demonstrated some harm.[51,52] Yet, there are case reports of dornase alfa in patients with ciliary dyskinesia that demonstrated benefit in some patients.[53] Similar to the results of aerosolized antibiotics in patients with non-CF bronchiectasis, these findings suggest that there are some patients with non-CF bronchiectasis who may benefit from such therapies, but the practice cannot be extrapolated to the entire population.

N-acetylcysteine (10–20% solution) has long been used as an aerosol medication with the attribution that it has mucolytic effects. However, there is no evidence to support such a mechanism, or that it improves clearance of airways secretions;[54] some have suggested that it may increase cough alone to account for any benefit. This approach to treatment has diminished in recent years, although there is a recent interest in whether N-acetylcysteine can be an immune modulator when given orally at pharmacologic doses.[55]

Hypertonic saline has been used with success in patients with CF with the proposed mechanism of temporarily replacing the volume of the airway surface liquid.[56] Although a diminished airway surface liquid is not the problem in most of the other types of non-CF bronchiectasis, hypertonic saline has also been used to increase ciliary clearance in this population.[57,58] It seems more likely that the added salt and water is able to modify the nature of the airway secretions making them easier to clear from the airways, or that hypertonic saline irritates the airways sufficiently to increase the cough clearance.

Anti-inflammatory Medications

Corticosteroids are commonly used to treat ABPA,[5,6] otherwise there are no randomized trials of systemic corticosteroids for non-CF bronchiectasis.[59] Inhaled corticosteroids are used widely in patients with CF and non-CF bronchiectasis without convincing evidence in the literature to support the practice. In a recent study, inhaled corticosteroids were withdrawn from patients with CF, with no detrimental effects found in the first six months;[60] although it could be argued as an insufficient period of time to know if inhaled corticosteroids can actually slow down the progression of disease. Inhaled corticosteroids for non-CF bronchiectasis have been shown to improve quality of life[61] and decrease 24-hour sputum volume,[62] but there are insufficient data to make any recommendation for their use.

High-dose ibuprofen has been studied in the CF population with the benefit of a slow rate of decline of FEV_1,[63] but this form of therapy has yet to be studied in non-CF bronchiectasis. Macrolide antibiotics have potent anti-inflammatory effects and have become increasingly popular in the treatment of patients with CF, and are being used with increased frequency in patients with non-CF bronchiectasis as well. The benefit of such therapy in patients with non-CF bronchiectasis is less clear, but small studies are encouraging.[64,65] However, chronic use of macrolides is strongly discouraged in patients with NTM present in sputum cultures, unless as a part of combination therapy for the treatment of NTM infection, to avoid the development of macrolide resistance.

WHAT IS AN EXACERBATION?

In general, a respiratory exacerbation is the worsening of respiratory symptoms (e.g., cough and sputum production) as well as some nonspecific systemic symptoms (e.g., decreased appetite) (Table 4-2). Attempts to define an exacerbation have been made,[52] and the signs and symptoms that are commonly reviewed in treatment of exacerbations include cough, sputum volume, changes in lung function (e.g., FEV_1), and exercise tolerance. Since some of the symptoms are present on a daily basis, it is important to determine how much they have changed. Cough is perhaps

Table 4-2	Signs and Symptoms of an Acute Exacerbation of Bronchiectasis[66]	
Increased cough	Fatigue, malaise
Increased sputum	Fever
Change in sputum (more purulent)	Radiographic changes (new pulmonary infiltrate)
Hemoptysis	
Change in exam (new crackles with or without wheeze)	Decreased pulmonary function measures

the most consistent finding and an instrument designed to assess the impact of cough severity is the Leicester Cough Questionnaire.[41] The 19-item survey provides an overall score in the range of 3–21 with a lower score correlating with greater severity of cough (severe 13.6, moderate 17.8, mild 19.3, $p < 0.0001$). When assessed at the diagnosis of an exacerbation in patients with bronchiectasis, the mean score was 11.3 and increased (i.e., less severe cough) to 17.8 at the completion of treatment. There may be fever or a reduction in pulmonary function as in patients with CF, but many patients will not experience a measureable change in FEV_1 likely because their sputum production is not as exaggerated as is seen in patients with CF. Likewise, the treatment of an exacerbation results in only a modest increase in FEV_1 (0.07 L, $p = 0.07$) primarily because most of the patients experienced either no or minimal improvement following treatment; only 19.3% realized at least a 12% or 200 mL increase in FEV_1.[41] The main improvement can be seen in a reduction in sputum volume and an increase in exercise tolerance.[41] Similarly, quality of life is worse during an acute exacerbation and improves with the treatment.[67]

Although there are not great changes in FEV_1 acutely, exacerbations are associated with a more rapid decline in lung function.[68] In this study, the average rate of loss of FEV_1 was 52.7 mL/year (or 2.35% predicted/year), much greater than a normal rate of change in FEV_1. A stepwise logistic regression determined the important factors associated with more rapid loss of lung function were the presence of *P. aeruginosa*, elevated C-reactive protein and severe exacerbations (defined as hospitalization, treatment with steroids, or respiratory failure).

CAUSES OF AN EXACERBATION

There is little knowledge about causes of an exacerbation in patients with non-CF bronchiectasis, but there is no reason to suspect that they would differ in comparison to those with CF (see Chapter 3 on CF). One must always consider a role for the underlying disease (e.g., ABPA), but many exacerbations are attributable to the bronchiectasis itself.

As antibiotics are commonly used to treat pulmonary exacerbations, it is presumed that the cause may involve either a new infection or a change in the chronic infection. Viral infection may be implicated and serologic testing may be necessary to establish the diagnosis. New bacteria may be introduced to the lower airways by aspiration. Similar to what has been proposed for CF, the bacteria chronically present in the airways may undergo a change, altering their virulence or numbers.[69] Aspiration, possibly associated with gastroesophageal reflux disease, may incite airways inflammation even in the absence of infection. Finally, environmental pollution could be shown to have an association with exacerbations as seen in CF.[70]

TREATMENT OF AN EXACERBATION

There are recently published guidelines on the treatment of acute pulmonary exacerbations for non-CF bronchiectasis.[38] The treatment of a non-CF pulmonary exacerbation is directed at the infection and inflammation, as well as the underlying disease process. It is advisable to continue with chronic medications and airway clearance therapies.

Site of Treatment

A decision must be made as to where the treatment of the exacerbation will take place, and this is typically based upon the perceived severity of disease. Oral antibiotics may be used to treat mild exacerbations in the home setting; and while intravenous antibiotics may also be delivered safely at home, this may not be an option or advisable for some patients. Other suggested criteria for inpatient treatment include an inability to take oral therapy, insufficient home resources or more severe illness (e.g., respiratory or circulatory failure).[38] Finally, some patients will be better served to be admitted to the hospital to focus on treatment components, such as airway clearance, that are critical to both short- and long-term treatment goals.

Antibiotics

As stated earlier, antibiotics are commonly used to treat exacerbations. The selected antibiotics may be delivered by the oral, inhaled, or intravenous routes. Although studies have not supported a benefit of aerosol therapies for chronic suppression in non-CF bronchiectasis, our knowledge of their use for acute exacerbations is limited.[71] Antibiotics are empirically selected based upon the results of previous sputum cultures. When these are not available, antibiotics should be selected to treat the most common pathogens (e.g., *H. influenzae, P. aeruginosa*). It is prudent to collect a new sputum culture at the time of diagnosis, so that the current culture data are available to guide therapy if the patient does not improve satisfactorily.

Combinations of antibiotics are frequently used to treat non-CF pulmonary exacerbations. As reviewed in the chapter on CF exacerbations, combinations of antibiotics are used to treat *Pseudomonas* infection even in the absence of clinical data to suggest that this strategy is necessary.[72] There is no compelling reason to believe that *Pseudomonas* would behave differently in non-CF pulmonary exacerbations,[38] yet combination antibiotics may be necessary for patients who have multiple bacterial species present in cultures.

Recommendations for dosing of antibiotics are described in table 4-3. Aerosol delivery of antibiotics results in high concentrations of drug in the airways, possibly

Table 4-3 Antibiotic Dosing Recommendations for Pulmonary Exacerbations of Bronchiectasis

Drugs	Pathogens*	Oral dosing	IV dosing	IV drug monitoring
Aminoglycosides				
Tobramycin	PA, HI		10 mg/kg/d divided every 12 h every 24 h	Peak 10–16 µg/mL Trough < 0.5 µg/mL Peak 25–35 µg/mL Trough < 0.5 µg/mL
Amikacin	PA, HI		30 mg/kg/d divided every 12 h every 24 h	Peak 15–20 µg/mL Trough < 5 µg/mL Peak 30–45 µg/mL Trough < 5 µg/mL
Penicillins				
Amoxicillin	MSSA	500 mg TID		
Piperacillin-tazobactam	PA, MSSA		4.5 g every 6 h	
Ticarcillin-clavulanate	PA, MSSA, SM		3.1 g every 4–6 h	
Cephalosporins				
Ceftazidime	PA, MSSA, HI		2 g every 8 h	
Cefepime	PA, MSSA, HI		2 g every 8 h	
Carbapenems				
Imipenem-cilastatin	PA, MSSA, HI		500 mg every 6 h	
Meropenem	PA, MSSA, HI		1–2 g every 8 h	
Doripenem	PA, MSSA, HI		500 mg every 8 h	
Monobactams				
Aztreonam	PA, MSSA, HI		2 g every 8 h	

Continued

Continued

Drugs	Pathogens*	Oral dosing	IV dosing	IV drug monitoring
Fluoroquinolones				
Ciprofloxacin	PA, MSSA, HI	500–750 mg BID–TID	400 mg TID	
Levofloxacin	PA, MSSA, HI, SM	750–1000 mg BID	750 mg every 12–24 h	
Moxifloxacin	PA, MSSA, HI, SM	400 mg BID	400 mg daily	
Tetracyclines				
Tigecycline	MSSA, MRSA		100 mg × 1, then 50 mg every 12 h	
Doxycycline	MSSA, MRSA, SM	100 mg BID	100 mg BID	
Minocycline	MSSA, MRSA, HI	200 mg, then 100 mg BID		
Others				
Vancomycin	MSSA, MRSA		15 mg/kg/d every 8–24 h	Trough 15–20 μg/mL
Linezolid	MSSA, MRSA	600 mg BID	600 mg BID	
Trimethoprim-Sulfamethoxazole	MSSA, MRSA, SM	15–20 mg/kg/d trimethoprim divided every 6 h	15–20 mg/kg/d trimethoprim divided every 6 h	
Colistin	PA		2 mg/kg every 12 h	
Chloramphenicol	HI, BC, SM		50–100 mg/kg/d divided every 6 h	Maximum 4–8 g/day

*The drugs generally have activity against these pathogens, but some organisms may be resistant.

PA, *Pseudomonas aeruginosa*; MSSA, methicillin-sensitive *Staphylococcus aureus*; MRSA, methicillin-resistant *Staphylococcus aureus*; HI, *Haemophilus influenzae*; SM, *Stenotrophomonas maltophilia*; BC, *Burkholderia cepacia*.

at the site of infection, but there are no studies that have compared aerosol to intravenous treatment of exacerbations, and aerosol antibiotics are not approved for the treatment of patients with non-CF bronchiectasis. Finally, there are no studies that have investigated the optimal duration of antibiotic therapy. The recently published guidelines suggested 14 days of treatment would be appropriate.[38]

Corticosteroids

Corticosteroids have been used to treat exacerbations of non-CF exacerbations as well. For the patients with ABPA, corticosteroids may be useful; otherwise, there are no randomized trials of systemic corticosteroids for non-CF bronchiectasis.[59] Inhaled corticosteroids are used widely in patients with CF and non-CF bronchiectasis without convincing evidence in the literature to support the practice. In a recent study, inhaled corticosteroids were withdrawn from patients with CF, with no detrimental effects found in the first six months;[60] although it could be argued that this is an insufficient period of time to know if inhaled corticosteroids can actually slow down the progression of disease. Inhaled corticosteroids for non-CF bronchiectasis have been shown to improve quality of life[61] and decrease 24-hour sputum volume,[62] but there are insufficient data to make any recommendation for their use. Other anti-inflammatory agents that have been used in patients with non-CF bronchiectasis include nonsteroidal anti-inflammatory drugs (NSAIDs), macrolides and leukotriene modifiers, but these would not be considered effective in the acute exacerbation. There is a growing evidence of benefit with chronic macrolides; although whether this is due to an antibacterial or anti-inflammatory effect, can be debated.[64,65]

COMPLICATIONS

There are other common pulmonary complications that are related to pulmonary exacerbations and warrant further discussion. For those patients with ABPA, an exacerbation in these patients could be due to the bronchiectasis or be a manifestation of allergic asthma. Hemoptysis occurs commonly as a part of pulmonary exacerbation and may be massive in amount. Respiratory failure is another manifestation of advanced lung disease and could be an aspect of a pulmonary exacerbation.

Allergic Bronchopulmonary Aspergillosis (ABPA)

The diagnosis and management of ABPA has been discussed earlier, but there are no specific features of disease that demonstrates when it is the allergic asthma that is the cause of an exacerbation. It may prove useful to measure an IgE level at the time of evaluation. Corticosteroid therapy is commonly used to treat ABPA exacerbations.[5,6]

Massive Hemoptysis

Fortunately, massive hemoptysis is a rare event but it can be life-threatening. The basic management of massive hemoptysis includes maintenance of the airway and a stable hemodynamic status. Thus, the patient must be able to clear the hemoptysis, but selective intubation may be necessary in some patients. Bronchial arterial embolization (BAE) has been used successfully in some patients.[73,74] There are no published guidelines on other aspects of management, but strategies are discussed in the chapter on CF exacerbations. As the hemoptysis may well be a manifestation of a pulmonary exacerbation, the patient should be treated with antibiotics. Airway clearance therapies should be stopped in the setting of massive hemoptysis. This is not because it is believed that airway clearance therapies cause hemoptysis, but they may impair clot formation and adherence resulting in more bleeding. Similarly, aerosol medications may be continued with the exception of hypertonic saline, again not because it caused the bleeding, but it may be irritating to the airways and can induce cough in some patients,[75] and possibly aggravates the hemoptysis. As for the CF patient, the patient with massive hemoptysis should not undergo bronchoscopy prior to BAE, as it offers little benefit and will delay performance of the procedure.

Surgery

Surgical resection has been performed for non-CF bronchiectasis for management of uncontrolled hemoptysis and persistent or recurring infection.[76-78] Although there are reports of clinical success, surgery is generally limited to specific patients, namely those with focal disease that can be completely resected and who can tolerate the operation.[38]

Respiratory Failure

There are few data on the natural history of non-CF bronchiectasis and its eventual progression to respiratory failure. There is no real difference in how to manage hypercapnic or hypoxic respiratory failure due to non-CF lung disease as compared to any other advanced stage obstructive airways disease. Oxygen supplementation is provided using the same parameters as for any other lung disease. Hypercapnic respiratory failure can be managed with ventilatory support, but intubation and mechanical ventilation for patients with advanced stage lung disease may have a poor prognosis; and for many patients, it is not an advisable treatment option unless they are listed for lung transplantation. Noninvasive ventilatory support using bi-level positive airway pressure (BiPAP) has been used with success as a palliative measure.[79-81]

CASE STUDY

A 67-year-old male with idiopathic bronchiectasis presents to clinic with complaints of increase in cough and sputum production over the last week. The sputum has become darker in color and there is a mild hemoptysis associated with the cough. There is no fever or chest pain. He feels more fatigued and there is an increment in his shortness of breath. His appetite is diminished and he feels that he may have lost weight.

On examination, he is afebrile; his weight is 62 kg, which is decreased from his baseline of 65 kg. Pulse oximetry reveals an arterial oxygen saturation of 94% on room air. His chest exam reveals crackles in both upper lung zones; these are unchanged from his previous exam. He has chronic clubbing to his fingers.

His current medications include albuterol by metered dose inhaled twice daily, hypertonic saline nebulized twice daily and azithromycin orally daily. His usual form of airway clearance therapy is oscillatory positive expiratory pressure using an Acapella device, but he admits that he has not been consistent with its use. His current spirometry measures are unchanged from his baseline measures (Figure 4-3). His current chest radiograph and a previous CT chest are shown in figure 4-4; there are no new findings.

The clinician makes the diagnosis of an acute pulmonary exacerbation and the decision is made to begin treatment in the hospital. He is started on ceftazidime and tobramycin based upon previous sputum cultures that have grown *P. aeruginosa* susceptible to these antibiotics. He is also started on his chronic

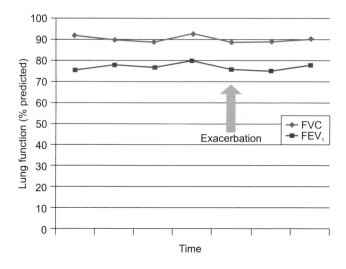

Figure 4-3 The results of spirometry.

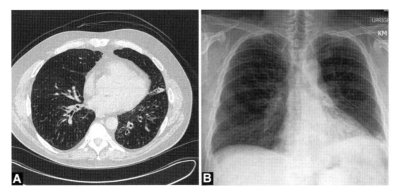

Figure 4-4 **A,** Baseline CT chest of patient. **B,** CXR of patient at the time of exacerbation.

therapies. Respiratory therapist begins chest physiotherapy and introduces him to high frequency chest compression.

After four days of therapy, the sputum culture obtained at admission has grown two strains of *P. aeruginosa,* both of which are susceptible to ceftazidime and tobramycin. The patient felt considerably better with less fatigue, a greater appetite, less cough and sputum production, and his hemoptysis resolved. The clinician decides to continue with the present therapy and on the fifth day, the patient is discharged from the hospital to complete a total of 14 days of intravenous antibiotics. At the completion of this therapy, the patient returns to clinic for removal of the PICC line and spirometry remains at the previous baseline (Figure 4-3).

CONCLUSION

The pulmonary exacerbation is a common event in the patient with non-CF lung bronchiectasis. It is generally believed that infection is a common factor in non-CF exacerbations and antibiotics have long been a standard approach to treatment. There are recently published guidelines on the diagnosis and management of non-CF bronchiectasis, but relatively few recommendations on the management of exacerbations. As for the CF pulmonary exacerbations, there is a great need to define best practices, so that we may optimize treatment and improve outcomes. To do so will require a standardized definition of an exacerbation. Ideally, the definition would be responsive to therapy, so we could assess acute therapies of exacerbations.

REFERENCES

1. Reid LM. Reduction in bronchial subdivision in bronchiectasis. *Thorax.* 1950;5:233-47.
2. Patel IS, Vlahos I, Wilkinson TM, et al. Bronchiectasis, exacerbation indices, and inflammation in chronic obstructive pulmonary disease. *Am J Respir Crit Care Med.* 2004; 170:400-7.

3. Weycker D, Edelsberg J, Oster G, et al. Prevalence and economic burden of bronchiectasis. *Clin Pulm Med.* 2005;12:205-9.

4. Cole PJ. Inflammation: A two-edged sword—the model of bronchiectasis. *Euro J Respir Dis Suppl.* 1986;147:6-15.

5. Moss RB. Pathophysiology and immunology of allergic bronchopulmonary aspergillosis. *Med Mycol.* 2005;43:S203-6.

6. Stevens DA, Moss RB, Kurup VP, et al. Allergic bronchopulmonary aspergillosis in cystic fibrosis—state of the art: Cystic Fibrosis Foundation Consensus Conference. *Clin Infect Dis.* 2003;37:S225-64.

7. Limper AH, Prakash UB. Tracheobronchial foreign bodies in adults. *Ann Inter Med.* 1990;112:604-9.

8. Kwon KY, Myers JL, Swensen SJ, et al. Middle lobe syndrome: a clinicopathological study of 21 patients. *Hum Pathol.* 1995;26:302-7.

9. Hornef N, Olbrich H, Horvath J, et al. DNAH5 mutations are a common cause of primary ciliary dyskinesia with outer dynein arm defects. *Am J Respir Crit Care Med.* 2006;174:120-6.

10. Noone PG, Leigh MW, Sannuti A, et al. Primary ciliary dyskinesia: diagnostic and phenotypic features. *Am J Respir Crit Care Med.* 2004;169:459-67.

11. Bush A, Chodhari R, Collins N, et al. Primary ciliary dyskinesia: current state of the art. *Arch Dis Child.* 2007;92:1136-40. (Epub 2007; July 18)

12. Reed W, Carson JL, Moats-Staats BM, et al. Characterization of an axonemal dynein heavy chain expressed early in airway epithelial ciliogenesis. *Am J Respir Cell Mol Biol.* 2000;23:734-41.

13. Driscoll JA, Bhalla S, Liapis H, et al. Autosomal dominant polycystic kidney disease is associated with an increased prevalence of radiographic bronchiectasis. *Chest.* 2008; 133:1181-8.

14. Edwards EA, Asher MI, Byrnes CA. Paediatric bronchiectasis in the twenty-first century: experience of a tertiary children's hospital in New Zealand. *J Paediatr Child Health.* 2003;39:111-7.

15. Pasteur MC, Helliwell SM, Houghton SJ, et al. An investigation into causative factors in patients with bronchiectasis. *Am J Respir Crit Care Med.* 2000;162:1277-84.

16. Reid KR, McKenzie FN, Menkis AH, et al. Importance of chronic aspiration in recipients of heart-lung transplants. *Lancet.* 1990;336:206-8.

17. Rosen FS, Cooper MD, Wedgwood RJ. The primary immunodeficiencies. *N Engl J Med.* 1995;333:431-40.

18. Eijkhout HW, van Der Meer JW, Kallenberg CG, et al. The effect of two different dosages of intravenous immunoglobulin on the incidence of recurrent infections in patients with primary hypogammaglobulinemia. A randomized, double-blind, multicenter crossover trial. *Ann Intern Med.* 2001;135:165-74.

19. Roifman CM, Levison H, Gelfand EW. High-dose versus low-dose intravenous immunoglobulin in hypogammaglobulinemia and chronic lung disease. *Lancet.* 1987;1:1075-7.

20. Bernatowska E, Madalinski K, Janowicz W, et al. Results of a prospective controlled two-dose crossover study with intravenous immunoglobulin and comparison (retrospective) with plasma treatment. *Clin Immunol Immunopathol.* 1987;43:153-62.

21. De Gracia J, Rodrigo MJ, Morell F, et al. IgG subclass deficiencies associated with bronchiectasis. *Am J Respir Crit Care Med.* 1996;153:650-5.

22. Hill SL, Mitchell JL, Burnett D, et al. IgG subclasses in the serum and sputum from patients with bronchiectasis. *Thorax.* 1998;53:463-8.

23. Buckley RH. Immunoglobulin G subclass deficiency: fact or fancy? *Curr Allergy Asthma Rep.* 2002;2:356-60.

24. McMahon MJ, Swinson DR, Shettar S, et al. Bronchiectasis and rheumatoid arthritis: a clinical study. *Ann Rheum Dis.* 1993;52:776-9.

25. Cortet B, Flipo RM, Remy-Jardin M, et al. Use of high resolution computed tomography of the lungs in patients with rheumatoid arthritis. *Ann Rheum Dis.* 1995;54:815-9.

26. Cohen M, Sahn SA. Bronchiectasis in systemic diseases. *Chest.* 1999;116:1063-74.

27. Angus RM, Davies ML, Cowan MD, et al. Computed tomographic scanning of the lung in patients with allergic bronchopulmonary aspergillosis and in asthmatic patients with a positive skin test to Aspergillus fumigatus. *Thorax.* 1994;49:586-9.

28. Mitchell TA, Hamilos DL, Lynch DA, et al. Distribution and severity of bronchiectasis in allergic bronchopulmonary aspergillosis (ABPA). *J Asthma.* 2000;37:65-72.

29. Hilliard T, Edwards S, Buchdahl R, et al. Voriconazole therapy in children with cystic fibrosis. *J Cyst Fibros.* 2005;4:215-20.

30. Zirbes JM, Milla CE. Steroid-sparing effect of omalizumab for allergic bronchopulmonary aspergillosis and cystic fibrosis. *Pediatr Pulmonol.* 2008;43:607-10.

31. Fowler SJ, French J, Screaton NJ, et al. Nontuberculous mycobacteria in bronchiectasis: Prevalence and patient characteristics. *Eur Respir J.* 2006;28:1204-10.

32. Wickremasinghe M, Ozerovitch LJ, Davies G, et al. Non-tuberculous mycobacteria in patients with bronchiectasis. *Thorax.* 2005;60:1045-51.

33. Salkin D. Tuberculosis as a cause of upper lobe bronchiectasis. *Calif Med.* 1950;73:577-80.

34. Newport MJ, Huxley CM, Huston S, et al. A mutation in the interferon-gamma-receptor gene and susceptibility to mycobacterial infection. *N Engl J Med.* 1996;335:1941-9.

35. Huang JH, Oefner PJ, Adi V, et al. Analyses of the NRAMP1 and IFN-gamma R1 genes in women with Mycobacterium avium-intracellulare pulmonary disease. *Am J Respir Crit Care Med.* 1998;157:377-81.

36. Olivier KN, Weber DJ, Wallace RJ, et al. Nontuberculous mycobacteria. I: multicenter prevalence study in cystic fibrosis. *Am J Respir Crit Care Med.* 2003;167:828-34.

37. Ziedalski TM, Kao PN, Henig NR, et al. Prospective analysis of cystic fibrosis transmembrane regulator mutations in adults with bronchiectasis or pulmonary nontuberculous mycobacterial infection. *Chest.* 2006;130:995-1002.

38. Pasteur MC, Bilton D, Hill AT, British Thoracic Society Bronchiectasis non-CFGG. British Thoracic Society guideline for non-CF bronchiectasis. *Thorax.* 2010;65:577.

39. Lynch DA, Newell J, Hale V, et al. Correlation of CT findings with clinical evaluations in 261 patients with symptomatic bronchiectasis. *Am J Roentgenol.* 1999;173:53-8.

40. Miszkiel KA, Wells AU, Rubens MB, et al. Effects of airway infection by *Pseudomonas aeruginosa:* a computed tomographic study. *Thorax.* 1997;52:260-4.

41. Murray MP, Turnbull K, MacQuarrie S, et al. Validation of the Leicester Cough Questionnaire in non-cystic fibrosis bronchiectasis. *Eur Respir J.* 2009;34:125-31.

42. Wilson CB, Jones PW, O'Leary CJ, et al. Validation of the St. George's Respiratory Questionnaire in bronchiectasis. *Am J Respir Crit Care Med.* 1997;156:536-41.

43. Wilson CB, Jones PW, O'Leary CJ, et al. Effect of sputum bacteriology on the quality of life of patients with bronchiectasis. *Eur Respir J.* 1997;10:1754-60.

44. Ho PL, Chan KN, Ip MS, et al. The effect of *Pseudomonas aeruginosa* infection on clinical parameters in steady-state bronchiectasis. *Chest.* 1998;114:1594-8.

45. Griffith DE, Aksamit T, Brown-Elliott BA, et al. An official ATS/IDSA statement: diagnosis, treatment, and prevention of nontuberculous mycobacterial diseases. *Am J Respir Crit Care Med.* 2007;175:367-416.

46. Flume PA, O'Sullivan BP, Robinson KA, et al. Cystic Fibrosis Pulmonary Guidelines: chronic medications for maintenance of lung health. *Am J Respir Crit Care Med.* 2007; 176:957-69.

47. Barker AF, Couch L, Fiel SB, et al. Tobramycin solution for inhalation reduces sputum *Pseudomonas aeruginosa* density in bronchiectasis. *Am J Respir Crit Care Med.* 2000; 162:481-5.

48. Scheinberg P, Shore E. A pilot study of the safety and efficacy of tobramycin solution for inhalation in patients with severe bronchiectasis. *Chest.* 2005;127:1420-6.

49. Eaton T, Young P, Zeng I, et al. A randomized evaluation of the acute efficacy, acceptability and tolerability of flutter and active cycle of breathing with and without postural drainage in non-cystic fibrosis bronchiectasis. *Chron Respir Dis.* 2007;4:23-30.

50. Fuchs HJ, Borowitz DS, Christiansen DH, et al. Effect of aerosolized recombinant human DNase on exacerbations of respiratory symptoms and on pulmonary function in patients with cystic fibrosis. The Pulmozyme Study Group.[comment]. *N Engl J Med.* 1994;331:637-42.

51. Wills PJ, Wodehouse T, Corkery K, et al. Short-term recombinant human DNase in bronchiectasis. Effect on clinical state and *in vitro* sputum transportability. *Am J Respir Crit Care Med.* 1996;154:413-7.

52. O'Donnell AE, Barker AF, Ilowite JS, et al. Treatment of idiopathic bronchiectasis with aerosolized recombinant human DNase I. rhDNase Study Group. *Chest.* 1998;113: 1329-34.

53. Desai M, Weller PH, Spencer DA. Clinical benefit from nebulized human recombinant DNase in Kartagener's syndrome. *Pediatr Pulmonol.* 1995;20:307-8.

54. Crockett AJ, Cranston JM, Latimer KM, et al. Mucolytics for bronchiectasis. [Update of Cochrane Database Syst Rev. 2000;(1):CD001289;PMID:10796636]. *Cochrane Database of Syst Rev.* 2001;(2):1.

55. Tirouvanziam R, Conrad CK, Bottiglieri T, et al. High-dose oral N-acetylcysteine, a glutathione prodrug, modulates inflammation in cystic fibrosis. Proceedings of the National Academy of Sciences of the United States of America 2006;103:4628-33.

56. Boucher RC. Evidence for airway surface dehydration as the initiating event in CF airway disease. *J Intern Med.* 2007;261:5-16.

57. Kellett F, Redfern J, Niven RM. Evaluation of nebulised hypertonic saline (7%) as an adjunct to physiotherapy in patients with stable bronchiectasis. *Respir Med.* 2005;99:27-31.

58. Wills PJ, Hall RL, Chan W, et al. Sodium chloride increases the ciliary transportability of cystic fibrosis and bronchiectasis sputum on the mucus-depleted bovine trachea. *J Clin Invest.* 1997;99:9-13.

59. Lasserson T, Holt K, Greenstone M. Oral steroids for bronchiectasis (stable and acute exacerbations). *Cochrane Database of Syst Rev.* 2001;(4):CD002162.

60. Balfour-Lynn IM, Lees B, Hall P, et al. Multicenter randomized controlled trial of withdrawal of inhaled corticosteroids in cystic fibrosis. *Am J Respir Crit Care Med.* 2006;173: 1356-62.

61. Martinez-Garcia MA, Perpina-Tordera M, Roman-Sanchez P, et al. Inhaled steroids improve quality of life in patients with steady-state bronchiectasis. *Respir Med.* 2006; 100:1623-32.

62. Tsang KW, Tan KC, Ho PL, et al. Inhaled fluticasone in bronchiectasis: a 12 month study. *Thorax.* 2005;60:239-43.

63. Konstan MW, Byard PJ, Hoppel CL, et al. Effect of high-dose ibuprofen in patients with cystic fibrosis. *N Engl J Med.* 1995;332:848-54.

64. Tsang KW, Ho PI, Chan KN, et al. A pilot study of low-dose erythromycin in bronchiectasis. *Eur Respir J.* 1999;13:361-4.

65. Cymbala AA, Edmonds LC, Bauer MA, et al. The disease-modifying effects of twice-weekly oral azithromycin in patients with bronchiectasis. *Treat Respir Med.* 2005;4: 117-22.

66. O'Donnell AE. Bronchiectasis. *Chest.* 2008;134:815-23.

67. Courtney JM, Kelly MG, Watt A, et al. Quality of life and inflammation in exacerbations of bronchiectasis. *Chron Respir Dis.* 2008;5:161-8.

68. Martinez-Garcia MA, Soler-Cataluna JJ, Perpina-Tordera M, et al. Factors associated with lung function decline in adult patients with stable non-cystic fibrosis bronchiectasis. *Chest.* 2007;132:1565-72.

69. VanDevanter DR, Van Dalfsen JM. How much do Pseudomonas biofilms contribute to symptoms of pulmonary exacerbation in cystic fibrosis? *Pediatr Pulmonol.* 2005;39: 504-6.

70. Goss CH, Newsom SA, Schildcrout JS, et al. Effect of ambient air pollution on pulmonary exacerbations and lung function in cystic fibrosis. *Am J Respir Crit Care Med.* 2004; 169:816-21.

71. Bilton D, Henig N, Morrissey B, et al. Addition of inhaled tobramycin to ciprofloxacin for acute exacerbations of *Pseudomonas aeruginosa* infection in adult bronchiectasis. *Chest.* 2006;130:1503-10.

72. VanDevanter DR. The value of *in vitro* susceptibility testing in guiding antibiotic choices for treatment of acute exacerbation. *Comment Chron Airways Infect.* 2007;2:8-13.

73. Rabkin JE, Astafjev VI, Gothman LN, et al. Transcatheter embolization in the management of pulmonary hemorrhage. *Radiology.* 1987;163:361-5.

74. Wong ML, Szkup P, Hopley MJ. Percutaneous embolotherapy for life-threatening hemoptysis. *Chest.* 2002;121:95-102.

75. Elkins MR, Bye PT. Inhaled hypertonic saline as a therapy for cystic fibrosis. *Curr Opin Pulm Med.* 2006;12:445-52.

76. Sanderson JM, Kennedy MC, Johnson MF, et al. Bronchiectasis: results of surgical and conservative management. A review of 393 cases. *Thorax.* 1974;29:407-16.

77. Prieto D, Bernardo J, Matos MJ, et al. Surgery for bronchiectasis. *Eur J Card Thora Surg.* 2001;20:19-23.

78. Balkanli K, Genc O, Dakak M, et al. Surgical management of bronchiectasis: analysis and short-term results in 238 patients. *Eur J Card Thora Surg.* 2003;24:699-702.

79. Benhamou D, Muir JF, Raspaud C, et al. Long-term efficiency of home nasal mask ventilation in patients with diffuse bronchiectasis and severe chronic respiratory failure: a case-control study. *Chest.* 1997;112:1259-66.

80. Dupont M, Gacouin A, Lena H, et al. Survival of patients with bronchiectasis after the first ICU stay for respiratory failure. *Chest.* 2004;125:1815-20.

81. Gacouin A, Desrues B, Lena H, et al. Long-term nasal intermittent positive pressure ventilation (NIPPV) in sixteen consecutive patients with bronchiectasis: a retrospective study. *Eur Respir J.* 1996;9:1246-50.

Acute Exacerbation of Idiopathic Pulmonary Fibrosis

Steven A Sahn

INTRODUCTION

Idiopathic pulmonary fibrosis (IPF) is a chronic, fibrosing, interstitial pneumonia of unknown cause.[1] It is limited to the lungs; and therefore, these patients do not present with or develop extrapulmonary manifestations as a direct consequence of IPF. The pleura is normal in IPF[2] and pleural effusions rarely occur in moderate-to-severe IPF, as the fibrosis in IPF is subpleural, preventing the movement of extravascular fluid from moving into the pleural space.

IDIOPATHIC INTERSTITIAL PNEUMONIAS (IIPs)

Incidence and Prevalence

IPF is the most common IIP, accounting for 47–63% of all IIP. Nonspecific interstitial pneumonia (NSIP) is the second most common with an incidence of 14–36%. Desquamative interstitial pneumonia (DIP) and respiratory bronchiolitis-associated ILD (RBILD) occur as a consequence of cigarette smoking and represent 0–16% of the cases of IIP. Cryptogenic organizing pneumonia has been reported in 6–7 per 1,00,000 hospital admissions. Acute interstitial pneumonia (AIP) was documented in 138 cases in 2003, representing 0–2% of the IIP. Lymphocytic interstitial pneumonia was reported in 13 patients at the Mayo Clinic over a 10-year period.[3-10]

Differentiating the IIPs

The various forms of IIP can be differentiated by patient demographics, physical examination, prodrome, treatment, prognosis, and ultimately histology. IPF is characterized by a chronic course, peripheral fibrosis, and honeycombing on high resolution computed tomography (HRCT) scan in a peripheral distribution with a basilar predominance, a poor response to treatment and a five-year, 50–70% mortality.[1,11] The pathology of IPF is usual interstitial pneumonia (UIP) with the hallmark of temporal heterogeneity, fibroblastic foci, and microscopic honeycombing.[1,12] In NSIP, there is subacute onset (months to years), peripheral, subpleural, basilar symmetric ground glass densities with or without pulmonary fibrosis in a basilar and peripheral distribution on HRCT scan; however, there is typically a clear separation between the ground glass opacities and fibrosis from the periphery of the lung.[1,10] The pathology of NSIP is diffuse, interstitial inflammation with or without fibrosis.[2,12] Cryptogenic organizing pneumonia typically presents in the fifth or sixth decade over a period of 2–3 months with malaise, fever, and other constitutional symptoms.[13] On HRCT of the chest, there are ground glass opacities, nodules, and consolidation; these lesions tend to be patchy and more prominent in the upper lung zones, involving the small airways and alveoli.[14,15] Pathology shows granulation tissue plugging alveolar ducts and alveoli.[16] Patients with AIP present over the age of 40 (mean 50–55) without gender predominance, as idiopathic ARDS with ground glass opacities and consolidation on HRCT scan in a diffuse, random distribution.[17,18] Pathology shows hyaline membranes, immature fibroblasts in the alveolar spaces and interstitium to a variable degree.[19] RB-ILD, probably more common in men, presents in the fourth or fifth decade with dyspnea and a multipack/year history of cigarette smoking. On HRCT scan, there are bronchiectasis and ground glass opacities in the upper lung zones in a bronchocentric distribution.[20] Pathology shows respiratory bronchiolitis surrounded by macrophages with a dusty-brown cytoplasm in the alveoli.[21] DIP presents with subacute dyspnea and cough, basilar crackles, and clubbing in up to 40% of patients. On HRCT, there are diffuse ground glass opacities and consolidation in a basilar, peripheral, and alveolar distribution.[22] Pathology demonstrates alveolar macrophages filling airspaces diffusely throughout the biopsy.[23] Lymphocytic interstitial pneumonia (LIP), more common in women, presents subacutely in the fourth to sixth decades with dyspnea and cough. On HRCT scan, there are ground glass opacities, nodules, and cysts in a patchy distribution.[24,25] An autoimmune pathogenesis of LIP is supported by the association with primary and secondary Sjögren's syndrome, pernicious anemia, myasthenia gravis, primary biliary cirrhosis, and chronic active hepatitis.[26]

EPIDEMIOLOGY OF IPF

It is estimated that the incidence of IPF is greater than 30,000 cases per year in the United States, with a prevalence estimated at more than 80,000.[27] However, these numbers are likely an underestimate, as a number of IPF patients are misdiagnosed as COPD or lung scarring by their primary care physicians. IPF is typically a disease of older individuals with the highest incidence and prevalence (1.5–1.7:1) occurring in males.[3,28] Approximately two-thirds of these patients are more than 60 years of age at the time of diagnosis.[13] However, the range of onset may be as young as 40 in a small percentage of individuals. Cigarette smoking is clearly a risk factor in patients with IPF, with about 70% being former or current smokers.[29,30] Familial IPF has been reported in a large number of case studies and is defined when two or more individuals with the entity are blood-related. Familial IPF is transmitted as an autosomal dominant trait with reduced penetrance and also tends to be more common in men.[31] Familial IPF has been reported in 0.5–2.2% of IPF cases in the United Kingdom[32] and 3.3–3.7% in Finland.[33] Possible, but not established, associated factors that may be causative in IPF include excessive exposure to wood or metal dust,[34,35] gastroesophageal reflux disease,[36] and infectious agents, predominantly viral infections. The role of viruses,[37] such as adenovirus, cytomegalovirus, influenza, hepatitis C,[38] or Epstein-Barr,[39] is unclear.

PATHOGENESIS

Patients who develop IPF have an abnormal response to injury, which is related to the inability to re-epithelialize the type-II pneumocytes and prevent the subsequent deposition of collagen, when injury occurs. As a possible explanation for the pathogenesis of IPF, Greider and Blackburn[40] reported that mutations occur and decrease the enzyme telomerase, which leads to ineffective regeneration of DNA and cell death. Telomerase has been implicated in several diseases, including a genetic disease, dyskeratosis congenita, with the telomerase mutation leading to lung fibrosis. These mutations result in shortened telomeres that are unable to repair the injury to the type-II alveolar cells leading to the uninhibited proliferation of myofibroblasts that promote collagen formation with each injury that occurs in the IPF patient. Telomerase mutations have been documented in 8% of patients with familial IPF. Genetics, telomerase mutations, cigarette smoke, toxins and oxidants through the environment and aging alone can result in abnormal telomeres with resultant impaired regenerative capacity of the epithelial cells and the development of fibrosis from mesenchymal cells.

CLINICAL PRESENTATION

Patients with IPF present most commonly in their 60s with chronic exertional dyspnea. The differential diagnosis of chronic exertional dyspnea includes, in additional to lung and cardiac disease, pulmonary vascular disease (such as pulmonary hypertension or arterial venous malformations), neuromuscular disease (including diaphragm dysfunction), and miscellaneous conditions (e.g., anemia, obesity, deconditioning, hyperthyroidism, and anxiety). The pulmonary differential diagnosis most commonly includes asthma, COPD, and interstitial lung disease. If the patient has basilar crackles, especially Velcro in character, IPF is most likely. A classic HRCT scan, interpreted by a trained observer, in the appropriate clinical setting (white male, age 65, former smoker), supports a confident clinical diagnosis of IPF in 90% of cases.[41] The median duration of illness prior to diagnosis is two years.[42] Clubbing occurs in 40–75% of patients who were most likely smokers.[42,43]

DIAGNOSIS OF IPF

The diagnostic criteria for IPF without a surgical lung biopsy include four major criteria: exclusion of other known causes of ILD; evidence of restriction with or without impaired gas exchange; HRCT scan showing peripheral, bibasilar, reticular abnormalities with minimal ground glass opacities; and transbronchial biopsies or bronchoalveolar lavage (BAL) that do not support an alternative diagnosis.

Minor criteria include: age > 50 years; the insidious onset of otherwise unexplained dyspnea on exertion; duration of illness greater than three months; and bibasilar Velcro crackles. All major criteria and at least three of the four minor criteria must be present to increase the likelihood of an IPF diagnosis.[1,2]

Excluding other conditions that can cause pulmonary fibrosis, such as connective tissue diseases (CTD), is of utmost importance in establishing the diagnosis of IPF.[44-49] Serologic tests that can help exclude an autoimmune disease include a normal or minimally elevated erythrocyte sedimentation rate, a negative or low titer ANA, a normal cyclic citrullinated peptide (CCP), a normal creatine kinase (CK) and aldolase, a negative extractable nuclear antigen (ENA) panel (Smith, RNP, SCL 70, SSA, and SSB antibodies) and a negative anti-myositis panel (including Jo-1).[49] A hypersensitivity pneumonitis panel should be obtained if there is a known exposure history such as birds in the home.

In patients with early IPF, the chest radiograph, HRCT scan, pulmonary function tests and resting ABG may be normal; and therefore, do not exclude the diagnosis of early IPF. Restriction may not always be present in patients with early disease. Classically, spirometry will show a reduced FVC and lung volumes a low TLC with a normal or increased FEV_1/FVC ratio in the nonsmoker or those with minimal smoking history. The primary cause of resting hypoxemia is a V/Q mismatch and does not result from either impaired oxygen diffusion or anatomic shunts.[50,51] Desaturation on a 6-MWT is a sensitive measure to evaluate impaired gas exchange in patients with IPF.[52,53]

If the patient presenting with interstitial lung disease is less than 50 years of age and has an atypical HRCT scan with increased ground glass density, mid-zone or upper lobe disease predominating over basilar disease or serology suggesting an autoimmune disease, the patient most likely does not have IPF. If autoimmune disease is not a consideration, then lung biopsy using video-assisted thoracoscopic surgery (VATS) should be strongly considered to establish the underlying cause of the interstitial lung disease.[54]

CLINICAL PREDICTORS OF SEVERITY AND PROGRESSION OF IPF

There are a number of prognostic factors that aid the clinician in the assessment of the IPF patient. These include baseline prognostic factors such as degree of dyspnea,[42,55,56] the degree of desaturation,[57-60] and distance traveled[61] on a 6-MWT and the arterial A-a O_2 gradient.[57,62] The HRCT pattern on chest imaging[63,64] and the histologic pattern[65,66] also provide prognostic information. In addition, the presence of pulmonary arterial hypertension[67-69] and neutrophilia on BAL[70] at baseline project a poor prognosis.

The causes of pulmonary hypertension are, most likely, multifactorial and include primary lesions of the vessels, compression and destruction of the pulmonary vessels by the interstitial process, vasoconstriction mediated by hypoxemia, acidemia pulmonary blood volume and a contribution from left ventricular dysfunction.

There are also several dynamic factors that are predictors of a worse outcome. These include the degree of dyspnea[42,57] and the decline in pulmonary function parameters such as the diffusion capacity (decline of > 15% over one year)[71] and the forced vital capacity (decline > 10% over six months).[57] An increase in the A-a O_2 gradient of > 15 mmHg also predicts a worse outcome.[57,62]

PROGNOSIS OF IPF

The survival of IPF from the time of diagnosis is generally considered to be 2–5 years; however, these figures are clearly affected by the timeliness of diagnosis. There are, however, factors both at the time of diagnosis and at follow-up that suggest a poor outcome. For example, the serum albumin concentration has been found to be a predictor of outcomes in patients with IPF.[72] As IPF becomes more advanced, depression often ensues and appetite is diminished. In a large multicenter study, it was found that those patients with albumin levels less than 3.3 g/dL had an adjusted hazard ratio of 5.8 as compared to those with an albumin of 4.6–5.3 g/dL, with an adjusted hazard ratio of 1.0.[72] Therefore, it is important to talk to patients about the importance of adequate nutrition, particularly protein intake. Any respiratory event that requires hospitalization predicts a worse survival.[73]

Patients with IPF should be monitored every 3–6 months with spirometry, diffusion, 6-MWT (6-minute walking test), and a quality of life questionnaire to assess dyspnea and to determine their oxygen requirements. An HRCT should only be repeated when there is an obvious clinical change. Comorbidities should be addressed at all routine visits. In a study of 110 patients with IPF, Patel and colleagues reported that 71% had comorbidities, most commonly GERD, hypertension, diabetes, and hypothyroidism.[74]

The course of the patient with IPF is characterized by the insidious progression of disease. However, the course of IPF is heterogeneous; and in a specific patient, it is problematic to predict the clinical outcome. A decrease in the FVC of up to 425 mL over a period of 72 weeks was documented in one of the capacity trials.[75] In addition, a decrease in the diffusion capacity of more than 15% over one year[71] or an FVC of more than 10% decline over six months[57] is termed as progression of disease and portends a worse prognosis. However, there are episodes of accelerated progression (acute exacerbation) which commonly lead to death or have a major negative impact on survival over the next several months.[76,77] An acute exacerbation of interstitial lung disease is not limited to IPF patients and has also been reported in patients with chronic hypersensitivity pneumonitis,[78,79] idiopathic NSIP, rheumatoid arthritis with UIP and scleroderma with NSIP.[80] However, far more cases of acute exacerbations have been reported in IPF compared to other interstitial lung diseases.

ACUTE EXACERBATION: A MISNOMER?

An acute exacerbation of IPF is actually a misnomer, as the typical presentation of this event is over a 1-4 weeks interval. According to standard and medical dictionaries, acute is defined, as related to health effect, as brief and not chronic, and is suggested to connote severe illness. Acute has also been defined as extremely severe, intense pain having a rapid onset and a short severe course. None of these terms appropriately define the presentation of an acute exacerbation of IPF; therefore, a more appropriate terminology for this entity should be a *subacute exacerbation* or an *accelerated phase of IPF.*

An accelerated phase of IPF does not occur over hours, or one or two days, but insidiously over a longer period of time with the following criteria: a known diagnosis of IPF; worsening of dyspnea of unknown cause over 1-4 weeks; new, bilateral ground glass densities or consolidation on a background of reticulation and honeycombing on HRCT scan; absence of infection on BAL or endotracheal aspirate; and exclusion of an alternate cause (such as infection, congestive heart failure, pulmonary embolism) or any known cause of acute lung injury (such as sepsis, gastric aspiration, fat embolism, pancreatitis, and others).[76,77]

Between 1987 and 2007, 20 series of patients with acute exacerbations of IPF were reported.[76] Of these 20 reports, five were case series, four were retrospective reviews of ICU admissions, two were retrospective reviews of post-lung biopsies, two were autopsy reviews, two were randomized control trials, two were retrospective reviews of lung biopsy cases, and one each was a retrospective review of hospital admissions, a retrospective cohort and a single survey.[76] The total number of patients reported in these 20 publications was 272, with a range of 3–51 patients per report. The mean age of these patients was 65.5 years with a range of 61–76 years of age. Males had a greater number of acute exacerbations, with a 4:1 male to female ratio. The mortality rate in the larger (9–22 patients) series ranged from 22 to 100%. The two year incidence of acute exacerbations was reported to be 9.6% in 11 patients. The three year incidence of the accelerated phase of IPF in 32 patients was 57%.[76]

An acute exacerbation may develop at any time during the course of IPF or may be the presenting manifestation. The severity of pulmonary function has not been correlated with the development of an acute exacerbation, as this entity has occurred over the entire spectrum of pulmonary function.[76,77] In addition, there appears to be no association with the patient's age or smoking history with the development of an acute exacerbation of IPF.[76] Possible precipitating factors that have been implicated in the development of an acute IPF exacerbation include an open lung biopsy,[81] bronchoalveolar lavage,[82] upper lobectomy, VATS lung biopsy, interferon-gamma therapy,[83] hypofractionated stereotactic body radiotherapy for lung cancer,[84] and *Chlamydia pneumoniae* infection. Martinez and colleagues[73] reported that 21% of 168 patients in the placebo group of an interferon-gamma trial over a period of 36 weeks died, and 47% of the deaths followed an acute deterioration. Kim and associates[85] reported a retrospective study of 147 patients with IPF proven by surgical lung biopsies; 11 (7.4%) had an acute exacerbation. The one and two years frequencies of acute exacerbations were 8.5% and 9.6%, respectively. Okamoto and others[86] reported an incidence of acute exacerbations at 25% over a 10 years period. Kubo and colleagues[87] reported the results of an anticoagulation trial from Japan; they found that 32 (57%) of 56 patients experienced an acute exacerbation. In a Japanese pirfenidone trial, Azuma and colleagues[88] reported a 14% (5/35) incidence of acute exacerbations in the placebo group compared to no acute exacerbations in the pirfenidone group.

Importantly, acute exacerbations of interstitial lung disease are not confined to the IPF population. These episodes of rapid acceleration of interstitial lung disease have been reported in NSIP, usually the idiopathic type and in others with connective tissue disease-associated ILD. Park and colleagues[80] reported a retrospective analysis of 74 patients with idiopathic NSIP and 93 patients with connective tissue associated interstitial lung disease. An acute exacerbation was reported in six (8.1%) of the patients with idiopathic NSIP with a one year frequency of 4.2%. Four (4.3%) individuals with a connective tissue-associated ILD (three with rheumatoid arthritis and one with scleroderma) had a one year frequency of acute exacerbation of 3.3%. These non-IPF patients with rapid deterioration of their disease tended to be younger than the IPF patients, with a median age of 58 years and a range of 47–75 years. Six (60%) of the 10 patients in the non-IPF series were women. Acute exacerbations occurred immediately following surgical lung biopsy and the median duration of acute symptoms prior to hospitalization for an acute exacerbation was 10 days, with a range of 1–30 days. The median PaO_2 as a fraction of the FIO_2 was 172, with a range of 107–273, with a PaO_2/FIO_2 ratio of < 200 in 6 of the 10 patients. A surgical lung biopsy, performed at the time of the acute exacerbation in two patients, revealed diffuse alveolar damage superimposed on an NSIP pattern.[80] Four patients with NSIP, idiopathic, survived to discharge and were evaluated at 6–21 months following the exacerbation. These data suggest that patients with NSIP, idiopathic, have a better prognosis following an acute exacerbation than those with IPF.

However, the three patients with rheumatoid-associated UIP had a poor outcome. The typical acute exacerbation in non-IPF patients is similar to the accelerated phase of IPF and is characterized by increasing dyspnea and worsening oxygenation over a 1–4 weeks period. Fever, cough, and flu-like symptoms have been recorded in some of these patients. There is typically severe gas exchange abnormalities with a PaO_2/FIO_2 ratio of < 225. These patients, more often than not, require noninvasive or mechanical ventilation. If BAL is performed, there will be a preponderance of neutrophils compatible with the findings in other forms of acute lung injury.

In a large series of patients with an acute exacerbation of IPF, an analysis of the HRCT data was reported in 2008.[89] There were 64 episodes of acute exacerbation in 58 IPF patients. The major findings in this study were typical features of IPF with superimposed, newly developed alveolar opacities; 34 (53%) patients had a peripheral pattern (Figure 5-1); 8 (12.5%) had a multifocal pattern (Figure 5-2A); and 16 (25%) had a diffuse pattern (Figure 5-2B); 25 (43.1%) of the 58 patients died and 33 (56.8%) survived following the initial exacerbation. Worse survival was associated with diffuse infiltrates compared to those with multifocal or peripheral infiltrates.[89] The CT patterns and overall CT content were associated with an increased likelihood of death after adjusting for age, gender, smoking, baseline diffusion capacity, baseline FVC, and disease extent on CT. On multivariate analysis, the strongest correlations were observed between CT patterns (combined diffuse and multifocal versus peripheral) and survival (odds ratio 4.6; 95% confidence interval, 1.90–11.28; P = 0.001).[89] This study suggests that CT assessment is potentially helpful in predicting patient prognosis following an acute exacerbation of IPF.

A decade prior, the same group reported CT findings in 17 patients with IPF who fulfilled the criteria for accelerated deterioration of disease.[90] Seven (70%) of

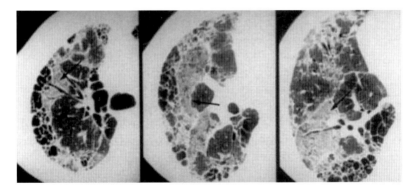

Figure 5-1 Peripheral pattern of acute exacerbation on HRCT scan. Note the peripheral areas of ground-glass attenuation adjacent to subpleural honeycombing. *From* Akira M, Hamada H, Sakatani M, et al. CT findings during the phase of accelerated deterioration in patients with idiopathic pulmonary fibrosis. *Am J Roentgenol.* 1997;168:79-83, with permission.

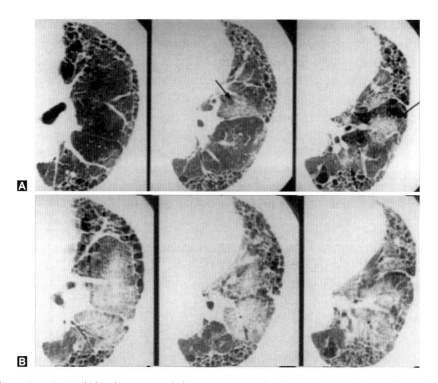

Figure 5-2 A, Multifocal pattern of the acute exacerbation on HRCT. Note the ground-glass opacities and consolidation at central and peripheral sites. **B,** Diffuse pattern of acute exacerbation on HRCT. Note the diffuse distribution of ground-glass opacities and subpleural honeycombing. *From* Akira M, Hamada H, Sakatani M, et al. CT findings during the phase of accelerated deterioration in patients with idiopathic pulmonary fibrosis. *Am J Roentgenol.* 1997;168:79-83, with permission.

the ten patients underwent sequential CT examinations and pathologic specimens were obtained from nine. Peripheral parenchymal calcifications were noted in six patients, multifocal parenchymal calcifications were seen in six patients, and diffuse parenchymal calcifications were seen in five. Multifocal lesions developed in two of the seven patients who had sequential CT scanning performed; these two patients died. Three of the six patients with a multifocal pattern responded to corticosteroid therapy. All patients with a peripheral pattern showed various degrees of improvement following corticosteroid therapy. Multifocal and diffuse parenchymal calcifications corresponded pathologically to acute and diffuse alveolar damage, while peripheral parenchymal calcifications corresponded pathologically to active fibroblastic foci. Akira and colleagues[90] concluded that HRCT patterns during periods of rapid deterioration in patients with IPF may provide a prediction of prognosis and response to treatment.

BIOMARKERS AND ACUTE EXACERBATIONS OF IPF

The pathobiology of an acute exacerbation of IPF has been extensively studied and encompasses injury to the alveolar epithelium, endothelial injury with increased vascular permeability, acute inflammation, and dysfunctional coagulation using plasma biomarkers, as a reflection of underlying abnormalities. Clinical studies of acute lung injury have defined a biological phenotype. Previously studied biomarkers of acute lung injury include KL-6,[91-93] surfactant protein D,[91-94] markers of type-II cell injury, a receptor for advanced glycation end-products (RAGE), a marker of type-I cell injury and proliferation,[95-97] and von Willebrand factor (vWF), a marker of endothelial cell injury.[98] Additional inflammatory markers also have been noted to be increased in acute lung injury, a reflection of the importance of acute inflammation in the development of this syndrome. Low levels of protein C and increased plasminogen activator inhibitor (PAI-1) have been well-documented coagulation abnormalities in acute lung injury. Collard and colleagues[99] recently reported the plasma biomarker profiles in patients with an acute exacerbation of IPF and compared them to the biomarkers in stable IPF. They found that plasma in patients with an acute exacerbation of IPF showed significant increase in markers of type-II alveolar epithelial cell injury, proliferation of endothelial cell injury, and coagulation. This profile differed from the biomarker profile when compared to those with acute lung injury in patients who did not have IPF. Their findings support the hypothesis that the type-II alveolar epithelial cells are centrally involved in the pathobiology of acute exacerbations of IPF. The data suggest that acute exacerbations of IPF have a distinct plasma biomarker profile compared to other forms of non-IPF, acute lung injury.

In the study by Collard and colleagues,[99] there were 20 patients with stable IPF, 47 patients with acute exacerbation of IPF, and 20 patients with non-IPF, acute lung injury. The mean age of all three groups ranged from 63 to 66 years. Approximately 80% were males, 90% had stable IPF, and 85% with an acute exacerbation of IPF were smokers. The patients with stable IPF had a mean FVC of 84% of predicted and those with acute exacerbations of IPF had an FVC of 75% of predicted. Four (20%) of the twenty patients with stable IPF were taking prednisone compared to 24 (51%) of 47 patients with an acute exacerbation of IPF who were receiving prednisone.

Exacerbations of IPF and non-IPF acute lung injury demonstrated strikingly different biomarker profiles. In acute exacerbations of IPF, the biomarker pattern suggested a relative predominance of type-II alveolar epithelial cell injury with or without proliferation and an absence of type-I alveolar epithelial cell activity compared to those patients who had non-IPF acute lung injury. The problematic issue in this study was the inability to document the precise time from the non-IPF acute lung injury to the blood draw compared to the known (18 days) interval in those with acute exacerbation of IPF. An unexpected finding was the increase in total protein C levels in acute exacerbations of IPF,[99] while in non-IPF, acute lung injury patients, the protein C levels were reduced; and in some cohorts, elevated levels of PAI-1 have been described.[100]

Except for thrombomodulin, no relationship between biomarker levels and short-term survival was noted in patients with acute exacerbation of IPF.[99] The significance of the association between survival and thrombomodulin is unclear.

Collard and associates[99] hypothesized that type-II alveolar epithelial cells are centrally involved in the pathobiology of acute exacerbations of IPF. Evidence is also provided for disordered coagulation. These data suggest that an acute exacerbation of IPF and non-IPF acute lung injury, while clinically similar, may be pathobiologically distinct. The authors suggest that future research should focus on the confirmation of the plasma biomarker profile and further characterization of the biology of the alveolar epithelial cell, endothelium and coagulation/fibrinolysis pathway in acute exacerbations of IPF. Studies that can find correlations of peripheral blood biomarker profiles with lung pathology in acute exacerbations of IPF may provide a new approach to the management of this lethal event in IPF patients.

Several hypotheses have been suggested as the cause of an acute exacerbation of IPF: a clinically occult condition that was undiagnosed, such as viral infection or gastric aspiration; a specific manifestation of the primary disease; or the sequelae of an acute, direct stress on the lung with an acceleration of the abnormal fibrinolytic response.[99,101-103] Loss of epithelial cell integrity, fibrocyte recruitment, MMP-9 and TGF-beta activation, disordered coagulation and fibrinolysis, and genetic predisposition all have been suggested as playing a role in this entity.[99-104] The inability to regenerate the epithelium of the type-II alveolar cells, which commonly occurs subclinically in IPF patients, may occur at a higher order of magnitude in acute exacerbations. It has recently been demonstrated that circulating fibrocytes are increased in the serum of IPF patients compared to controls in acute exacerbations, and the level of fibrocytes has been noted to be increased to a greater percentage.[105] Fibrocytes, bone marrow-derived mesenchymal precursor cells, may potentiate fibrogenesis through the generation of profibrotic factors.[106] Matrix metalloproteases, such as MMP-9, regulate extracellular matrix protein turnover and have been documented to be increased in BAL fluid of IPF patients.[107] Their role may be to promote the disruption of the functional integrity of the alveolar capillary membrane and to enhance the activation of TGF-beta.[108] Disordered coagulation or fibrinolysis may occur in acute exacerbations of IPF.[109] Lastly, patients with IPF may have a genetic predisposition to develop acute exacerbations. For example, the presence of mutations in the telomerase reverse transcriptase (hTERT) and the RNA component (hTR) genes encoding telomerase components have been reported in families with IPF.[110] Importantly, these mutations may be the cause of shortened telomeres that limit the regeneration of the alveolar epithelial cells.[111]

MANAGEMENT OF THE ACUTE EXACERBATION

Currently, there are no data from randomized controled trials to guide clinicians in managing patients with an acute exacerbation of IPF. Most authors report that treatment with high-dose corticosteroids, full spectrum antibiotics, cyclosporin,[112-114] and cyclophosphamide have been used without strong evidence of benefit. However, a single study showed that cyclosporin, after treatment with corticosteroids, increased survival (up to 208 weeks) as compared to corticosteroids alone (66 weeks).[112] The rationale for corticosteroid usage may be for the treatment of an organizing pneumonia; where the misdiagnosis, without treatment, could be disastrous to the patient. It is possible that anticoagulation may be helpful in these patients. In an open label study from Japan, 56 patients were randomized to prednisone plus warfarin (n = 23) or prednisone alone[33] over a period of three years.[87] The warfarin group had a lower mortality rate and decreased incidence of acute exacerbation compared to the control population. However, the study had flaws that prevented definitive conclusions such as nonblinding and a significant dropout rate. In a small (n = 107) pirfenidone trial in Japan, all exacerbations 5/35 (14%) occurred in the placebo group; and the study was subsequently discontinued after the DMSB recommendation.[88] However, this finding was not confirmed in a larger, follow-up, phase-III, pirfenidone trial in Japan.[115]

Song and colleagues recently reported a retrospective review of 461 patients with IPF (269 with biopsy proven disease) to estimate the incidence, risk factors and impact of acute exacerbations, and other known causes of rapid deterioration.[116] The median follow-up of these 461 patients was 22.9 months. Rapid deterioration requiring hospitalization occurred in 163 (35.4%) of these patients, with multiple episodes in 42 patients. Acute exacerbation was the most frequent cause of hospitalization occurring in 55.2%, followed by infection. The one year and three years incidences of acute exacerbation were 14.2, and 20.7%, respectively. Being never a smoker and having a low forced vital capacity (FVC) were significant risk factors for acute exacerbation. The in-hospital mortality was 50% and the 1–5 years survival rates from the initial diagnosis were from 56.2 to 18.4%. Acute exacerbation was a significant predictor of poor survival after the initial diagnosis, along with increased age, low FVC and diffusion capacity, and corticosteroid usage with or without cytotoxic therapy.

ICU Outcomes

In a retrospective analysis of 38 patients with IPF who were admitted to an ICU, 20 (53%) were receiving corticosteroids at the time of admission and 24 (63%) were using home oxygen.[117] The acute physiology and chronic health evaluation III (APACHE III) scores predicted ICU hospital mortality rates of 12% and 26%; and the actual ICU and hospital mortality rates were 45% and 61%, respectively. The investigators

CASE STUDY

A 61-year-old Caucasian male was initially diagnosed with IPF in 2006 by his clinical presentation and a video-assisted thoracoscopic lung biopsy. He was a former smoker and had minimal GERD symptoms at presentation. He denied significant occupational exposure, such as asbestos or wood or metal dust, and denied ever having birds in his home. There was no familial history of IPF and no history compatible with connective tissue disease in his family or symptoms suggestive of a connective tissue disease.

On physical examination, the patient was an overweight man who showed no evidence of increased work of breathing on room air. He was normotensive with a regular heart rate of 82 beats/minute. His weight was 203 pounds with a height of 69 inches. Room air oxygen saturation at rest was 94%. Lung examination revealed bibasilar and biaxillary velcro crackles with normal breath sounds heard over the upper lung zones. There was no clubbing of the digits and no peripheral edema was present.

Spirometry at presentation revealed an FVC of 65% of predicted with an FEV_1/FVC ratio of 85%. Total lung capacity was 60% of predicted, and the diffusion capacity was 55% of predicted. A room air ABG showed pH 7.44, PCO_2 33 mmHg, and PO_2 80 mmHg. On a 6-MWT, he walked a distance of 1300 ft with desaturation to 90% on room air. On echocardiogram, the left ventricular ejection fraction was estimated to be at 60%. The left atrial size was normal, and the right atrium and right ventricle were normal in size. The RVSP was estimated to be 28 mmHg. HRCT showed a typical pattern virtually diagnostic of IPF.

He received treatment by an outside physician in mid-2007 with prednisone, azathioprine, and n-acetyl cysteine (NAC). However, over the next several weeks, his pulmonary function deteriorated and he desaturated on a 6-MWT to a nadir of 83%. Over the next two months, his condition stabilized with minimal change in pulmonary function testing and no significant change in his dyspnea with exertion. A repeat echocardiogram now showed an RVSP of 40 mmHg and the patient was started on Bosentan without improvement; the drug was discontinued two months later.

He subsequently presented two years following his diagnosis with worsening dyspnea at rest that developed over a two-week period. He denied fever, chill, or night sweats. He was admitted to a local hospital with an oxygen saturation of 90-91% on 6 L/min of nasal cannula oxygen and BIPAP was instituted. In hospital, he remained afebrile, and blood and sputum cultures were negative. An HRCT scan (Figure 5-3A to D) with contrast showed new bilateral alveolar infiltrates on a background of a UIP pattern and no evidence of pulmonary emboli was found. He was subsequently treated with high-dose corticosteroids, diuretics, and broad-spectrum antibiotic coverage. After discussion with the family, he was intubated and placed on mechanical ventilation. BAL showed a neutrophil predominance

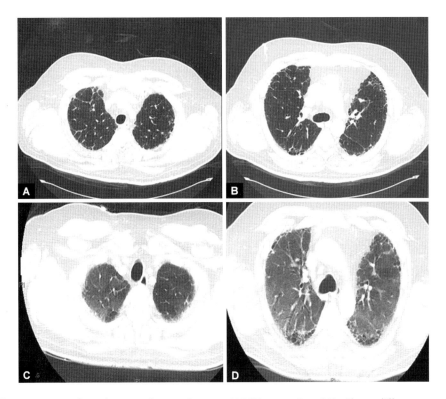

Figure 5-3 **A and B,** Show evidence of IPF on HRCT scan. **C and D,** Show diffuse ground-glass densities over the upper and lower lung zones compatible with an acute exacerbation of IPF.

and no evidence of pulmonary hemorrhage. The patient was evaluated for lung transplantation. Forty-eight hours later, the evaluation was completed; and 24 hours thereafter, a double lung transplant was performed. The patient was extubated on postoperative day two and was on room air on postoperative day five and did not require supplementary oxygen thereafter. He returned to work after of six months following transplantation.

As has previously been discussed in the text of this manuscript, the outcome of acute exacerbation of patients with IPF is generally poor, with a mortality rate over several months approaching 70%. This patient was a prototypic patient to develop IPF, an older male with an FVC of 55% of predicted. He had the classic HRCT of an acute exacerbation of IPF. As was discussed with the patient and his family, the need for mechanical ventilation to prolong survival was imminent, and the patient and his family decided to pursue lung transplantation. At the time of writing this report, the patient continues to do well, 18 months post-transplant.

found no significant difference in pulmonary function or echocardiogram findings between survivors and nonsurvivors. Mechanical ventilation was instituted in 19 (50%) of these patients. Ninety-two percent of the hospital survivors died within two months following discharge. Other smaller series support the ICU and post-ICU outcomes of these patients.[117-120] These results suggest that IPF patients admitted to the ICU have an extremely poor, short- and long-term prognosis. Therefore, patients with IPF and their families should be informed of this posibility, when decisions are made about life support and ICU care. This information is also applicable to IPF patients who have an acute exacerbation. With these factors in mind, a trial of mechanical ventilation with supportive care, corticosteroids, and broad-spectrum antibiotics is reasonable; however, if recovery does not appear imminent and lung transplantation is not an option, life support should be withdrawn with professionalism and dignity at the appropriate time for the patient and their family.

CONCLUSION

It is evident that an acute exacerbation is a manifestation of IPF that cannot be predicted, based on the severity of disease. However, this entity appears to be more common in elderly men, with no known precipitating factors and an FVC in the range of 50–80% of predicted. It is currently unknown whether an acute exacerbation is simply a variant of the underlying disease or is caused by a distinct process such as occult infection or gastric aspiration. A better understanding of this entity requires cooperation from clinicians involved in the care of IPF patients to combine their data in a prospective registry, documenting all pertinent information. The registry should include, not only clinical data, but a study of biomarkers that can predict the onset of these exacerbations and provide further insight into the pathobiology and treatment of this lethal entity.

REFERENCES

1. Travis WD, King TE Jr, Bateman ED, et al. American Thoracic Society/European Respiratory Society International multidisciplinary Consensus Classification of the Idiopathic Interstitial Pneumonias. *Am J Respir Crit Care Med.* 2002;165:277-304.
2. English JC, Leslie KO. Pathology of the pleura. *Clinics Chest Med.* 2006;27:157-80.
3. Coultas DB, Zumwalt RE, Black WC, Sobonya RE. The epidemiology of interstitial lung disease. *Am J Respir Crit Care Med.* 1994;150:967-72.
4. Chan-Yeung M, Muller NL. Cryptogenic fibrosing alveolitis. *Lancet.* 1997;350:651-6.
5. Bjoraker JA, Ryu JH, Edwin MK, et al. Prognostic significance of histopathologic subsets in idiopathic pulmonary fibrosis. *Am J Respir Crit Care Med.* 1998;157:199-203.
6. Nagai S, Kitachi M, Iroh H, et al. Idiopathic, nonspecific interstitial pneumonia/fibrosis: comparison with idiopathic pulmonary fibrosis and BOOP. *Eur Respir J.* 1998;12:1010-19.
7. Travis WD, Matsui K, Moss J, Ferrans VJ. Idiopathic non-specific interstitial pneumonia: Prognostic significance of cellular and fibrosing patterns: survival comparison with

usual interstitial pneumonia and desquamative interstitial pneumonia. *Am J Surg Pathol.* 2000;24:19-33.

8. Nicholson AG, Colby TV, du Bois RM, et al. The prognostic significance of histologic pattern of interstitial pneumonia in patients presenting with the clinical entity of cryptogenic fibrosing alveolitis. *Am J Respir Crit Care Med.* 2000;162:2213-7.

9. Park CS, Chung SW, Ki SY, et al. Increased levels of interleukin-6 are associated with lymphocytosis in bronchioalveolar lavage fluids of idiopathic, nonspecific interstitial pneumonia. *Am J Respir Crit Care Med.* 2000;162:1162-8.

10. Flaherty KR, Toews GB, Travis WD, et al. Clinical significance of histologic classification of idiopathic interstitial pneumonia. *Eur Respir J.* 2002;19:275-83.

11. King TE Jr, Costabel U, Cordier JF, et al. Idiopathic pulmonary fibrosis: diagnosis and treatment. International consensus statement. American Thoracic Society (ATS) and the European Respiratory Society (ERS). *Am J Respir Crit Care Med.* 2000;161:646-64.

12. Katzenstein AL, Myers JL. Idiopathic pulmonary fibrosis: clinical relevance of pathologic classification. *Am J Respir Crit Care Med.* 1998;157:1301-15.

13. Cordier JF. Organizing pneumonia. *Thorax.* 2000;55:318-28.

14. Bouchardy LM, Kuhlman JE, Ball WC Jr, et al. CT findings in bronchiolitis obliterans organizing pneumonia (BOOP) with radiographic, clinical, and histologic correlation. *J Comput Assist Tomogr.* 1993;17:352-7.

15. Preidler KW, Szolar DM, Moelleken S, et al. Distribution pattern of computed tomography findings in patients with bronchiolitis obliterans organizing pneumonia. *Invest Radiol.* 1996;31:251-5.

16. Colby TV, Myers JL. The clinical and histologic spectrum of bronchiolitis obliterans including bronchiolitis obliterans organizing pneumonia (BOOP). *Semin Respir Med.* 1992;13:119-33.

17. Ichikado K, Johkoh T, Ikezoe J, et al. Acute interstitial pneumonia: high-resolution CT findings correlated with pathology. *Am J Roentgenol.* 1997;168:333-8.

18. Hansell DM. Acute interstitial pneumonia: clues from the white stuff. *Am J Respir Crit Care Med.* 2002;165:1465-6.

19. Katzenstein ALA, Myers JL, Mazur MT. Acute interstitial pneumonia. A clinic pathologic, ultrastructural, and cell kinetic study. *Am J Surg Pathol.* 1986;10:256-67.

20. Park JS, Brown KK, Tuder RM, et al. Respiratory bronchiolitis-associated interstitial lung disease: radiologic features with clinical and pathologic correlation. *J Comput Assist Tomogr.* 2002;26:13-20.

21. Yousem SA, Colby TV, Gaenslar EA. Respiratory bronchiolitis-associated interstitial lung disease and its relationship to desquamative interstitial pneumonia. *Mayo Clin Proc.* 1989;64:1373-80.

22. Hartman TE, Primack SL, Swensen SJ, et al. Desquamative intersitial pneumonia: thin-section CT findings in 22 patients. *Radiology.* 1993;187:787-90.

23. Liebow AA, Steer A, Billingsley JG. Desquamative intersitial pneumonia. *Am J Med.* 1965;39:369-404.

24. Strimlan C, Rosenow EI, Weiland L, et al. Lymphocytic interstitial pneumonitis: a review of 13 cases. *Ann Intern Med.* 1978;68:616-21.

25. Johkoh T, Muller NL, Pickford HA, et al. Lymphocytic interstitial pneumonia: thin-section CT findings in 22 patients. *Radiology.* 1999;212:567-72.

26. Levinson A, Hopewell P, Steites D, et al. Co-existent lymphoid interstitial pneumonia, pernicious anemia, and agammaglobulinemia: common autoimmune pathogenesis. *Arch Intern Med.* 1976;136:213-6.

27. Raghu G, Weycher D, Edelsberg J, et al. Incidence and prevalence of idiopathic pulmonary fibrosis. *Am J Respir Crit Care Med.* 2006;174:810-6.

28. Coultas DB. Epidemiology of idiopathic pulmonary fibrosis. *Semin Respir Med.* 1993; 14:181-96.

29. Baumgartner KB, Samat J, Stidley CA, et al. Cigarette smoking: a risk factor for idiopathic pulmonary fibrosis. *Am J Respir Crit Care Med.* 1997;155:242-8.

30. Johnston ID, Prescott RJ, Chalmers JC, Rudd RM. British Thoracic Society study of cryptogenic fibrosing alveolitis: current presentation and initial management. Fibrosing Alveolitis Subcommittee of the Research Committee of the British Thoracic Society. *Thorax.* 1997;52:38-44.

31. Peabody JW, Peabody JW Jr, Hayes EW, et al. Idiopathic pulmonary fibrosis; its occurrence in identical twin sisters. *Dis Chest.* 1950;18:330-44.

32. Marshall RP, Puddicombe A, Cookson WO, Laurent GJ. Adult, familial, cryptogenic fibrosing alveolitis in the United Kingdom. *Thorax.* 2000;55:143-6.

33. Hodgson U, Laitmen T, Tukainen P. Nationwide prevalence of sporadic and familial idiopathic pulmonary fibrosis: evidence of founder effect among multiplex families in Finland. *Thorax.* 2002;57:338-42.

34. Hubbard R, Lewis S, Richards K, et al. Occupational exposure to metal or wood dust and aetiology of cryptogenic fibrosing alveolitis. *Lancet.* 1996;347:284-9.

35. Mapel DW, Coultas DB. The environmental epidemiology of idiopathic interstitial lung disease, including sarcoidosis. *Semin Respir Crit Care Med.* 1999;20:521-9.

36. Tobin RW, Pope CE II, Pellegrini CA, et al. Increased prevalence of gastroesophageal reflux in patients with idiopathic pulmonary fibrosis. *Am J Respir Crit Care Med.* 1998; 158:1804-8.

37. Egan JJ, Woodcock AA, Stewart JP. Viruses and idiopathic pulmonary fibrosis. *Eur Respir J.* 1997;10:1433-7.

38. Irving WL, Day S, Johnston ID. Idiopathic pulmonary fibrosis and hepatitis C virus infection. *Am Rev Respir Dis.* 1993;148:1683-4.

39. Egan JJ, Stewart JP, Hasleton PS, et al. Epstein-Barr virus replication within pulmonary epithelial cells in cryptogenic fibrosing alveolitis. *Thorax.* 1995;50:1234-9.

40. Greider CW, Blackburn EH. Telomeres, telomerase, and cancer. *Scientific Am.* 1996; 274:92-6.

41. Tung KT, Wells AU, Rubens MB, et al. Accuracy of the typical computed tomographic appearances of fibrosing alveolitis. *Thorax.* 1993;48:334-8.

42. King TE Jr, Tooze JA, Schwarz MI, et al. Predicting survival in idiopathic pulmonary fibrosis: scoring system and survival model. *Am J Respir Crit Care Med.* 2001;164: 1171-81.

43. Turner-Warwick M, Burrows B, Johnson A. Cryptogenic fibrosing alveolitis: clinical features and their influence on survival. *Thorax.* 1980;35:171-80.

44. Turner-Warwick M. Immunologic aspects of systemic diseases of the lung. *Proc R Soc Med.* 1974;67:541-7.

45. Salaffi F, Manganelli P, Carotti M, et al. The differing patterns of subclinical pulmonary involvement in connective tissue diseases as shown by application of factor analysis. *Clin Rheumatol.* 2000;19:35-41.

46. Sahn SA. Pathogenesis of pleural effusions and pleural lesions. In: Cannon GW, Zimmerman GA (Eds): *The Lung in Rheumatic Disease.* New York: Marcel Dekker; 1990. pp 27-45.

47. Sahn SA. Pathophysiology of pleural effusions. *Annu Rev Med.* 1990;41:7-13.

48. Ferri C, Valentini G, Cozzi F, et al. Systemic sclerosis: demographic, clinical, and serologic features and survival in 1,012 Italian patients. *Medicine.* 2002;81:139-53.

49. Kalluri M, Sahn SA, Oddis CV, et al. Clinical profile of anti-PL-12 autoantibody: cohort study and review of the literature. *Chest.* 2009;135:1550-6. Epub 2009 Feb 18. Review.

50. Austrian R, McClement JH, Renzetti AD Jr, et al. Clinical and physiologic features of some types of pulmonary diseases with impairment of alveolar capillary diffusion: the syndrome of alveolar-capillary blocks. *Am J Med.* 1951;11:667-85.

51. Holland RA, Blacket RB. Pulmonary function in the Hamman-Rich syndrome: the abnormalities of ventilation, blood gasses, and diffusion at rest and on exercise. *Am J Med.* 1960;29:955-66.

52. Sue DY, Oren A, Hansen JE, et al. Diffusion capacity of carbon monoxide as a predictor of gas exchange during exercise. *N Engl J Med.* 1987;316:1301-6.

53. Agusti AG, Roca J, Gea J, et al. Mechanisms of the gas-exchange impairment in idiopathic pulmonary fibrosis. *Am Rev Respir Dis.* 1991;143:219-25.

54. Krassner MJ, White CS, Aisner SC, et al. The role of thoracoscopy in the diagnosis of interstitial lung disease. *Ann Thorac Surg.* 1995;59:348-51.

55. Papiris SA, Daniil ZD, Malagari K, et al. The Medical Research Council Dyspnea Scale and the estimation of disease severity in idiopathic pulmonary fibrosis. *Respir Med.* 2005; 99:755-61.

56. Mogulkoc N, Brutsche MH, Bishop PW, et al. Pulmonary function in idiopathic pulmonary fibrosis and referral for lung transplantation. *Am J Respir Crit Care Med.* 2001;164:103-8.

57. Collard HR, King TE Jr, Bartelson BB, et al. Changes in clinical and physiologic variables predict survival in idiopathic pulmonary fibrosis. *Am J Respir Crit Care Med.* 2003;168: 538-42.

58. Lama VN, Flaherty KR, Toews GB, et al. Prognostic value of desaturation during a 6 MWT in idiopathic pulmonary fibrosis. *Am J Respir Crit Care Med.* 2003;168:1084-90.

59. Eaton T, Young P, Milne D, et al. Wells six-minute walk, maximal exercise tests reproducibility in fibrotic interstitial pneumonia. *Am J Respir Crit Care Med.* 2005;171: 1150-57.

60. Flaherty KR, Andrei AC, Murray S, et al. Idiopathic pulmonary fibrosis: prognostic value of changes in physiology and six-minute-walk test. *Am J Respir Crit Care Med.* 2006;174:803-9.

61. Lederer DJ, Arcasoy SM, Wilt JS, et al. Six-minute-walk distance predicts waiting list survival in idiopathic pulmonary fibrosis. *Am J Respir Crit Care Med.* 2006;174:659-64.

62. King TE Jr, Safrin S, Starko KM, et al. Analyses of efficacy end points in a controlled trial of interferon-gamma-lb for idiopathic pulmonary fibrosis. *Chest.* 2005;127:171-7.

63. Lynch DA, Godwin JD, Safrin S, et al. High-resolution computed tomography in idiopathic pulmonary fibrosis: Diagnosis and prognosis. *Am J Respir Crit Care Med.* 2005;172: 488-93.

64. Flaherty KR, Thwaite EL, Kazerooni EA, et al. Radiological versus histological diagnosis in UIP and NSIP: Survival implications. *Thorax.* 2003;58:143-8.

65. King TE Jr, Schwarz MI, Brown K, et al. Idiopathic pulmonary fibrosis: relationship between histopathologic features and mortality. *Am J Respir Crit Care Med.* 2001;164: 1025-32.

66. Nicholson AG, Fulfrod LG, Colby TV, et al. The relationship between individual histologic features and disease progression in idiopathic pulmonary fibrosis. *Am J Respir Crit Care Med.* 2002;166:173-7.

67. Lettieri CJ, Nathan SD, Barnett SD, et al. Prevalence and outcomes of pulmonary arterial hypertension in advanced idiopathic pulmonary fibrosis. *Chest.* 2006;129:746-52.

68. Hamada K, Nagai S, Tanaka S. Significance of pulmonary arterial pressure and diffusion capacity of the lung as prognosticator in patients with idiopathic pulmonary fibrosis. *Chest.* 2007;131:650-6.

69. Nathan SD, Shlobin OA, Ahmad S, et al. Pulmonary hypertension and pulmonary function testing in idiopathic pulmonary fibrosis. *Chest.* 2007;131:657-63.

70. Kinder BW, Brown KK, Schwarz MI, et al. Baseline BAL neutrophilia predicts early mortality in idiopathic pulmonary fibrosis. *Chest.* 2008;133:226-32.

71. Latsi PI, du Bois RM, Nicholson AG, et al. Fibrotic idiopathic interstitial pneumonia: the prognostic value of longitudinal functional trends. *Am J Respir Crit Care Med.* 2003;168:531-7.

72. Zisman DA, Kawut SM, Lederer DJ, et al. Serum albumin concentration and waiting list mortality in idiopathic interstitial pneumonia. *Chest.* 2009;135:929-35.

73. Martinez FJ, Safrin S, Weycker D, et al. The clinical course of patients with idiopathic pulmonary fibrosis. *Ann Intern Med.* 2005;142:963-7.

74. Patel S, Takahashi S, Demchuk C, et al. Gastroesophageal reflux disease in patients with idiopathic pulmonary fibrosis. *Am J Respir Crit Care Med.* 2009;179:A4063.

75. Noble PW, Albera C, Bradford WZ, et al. The CAPACITY Program: two randomized, double-blind, placebo-controlled trials of pirfenidone in patients with idiopathic pulmonary fibrosis. *Lancet* (in press).

76. Collard HR, Moore BB, Flaherty KR, et al. Acute exacerbations of idiopathic pulmonary fibrosis. *Am J Respir Crit Care Med.* 2007;176:636-43.

77. Agarwal R, Jindal SK. Acute exacerbations of idiopathic pulmonary fibrosis: a systematic review. *Eur J Intern Med.* 2008;19:227-35.

78. Olson AL, Huie TJ, Groshong SD, et al. Acute exacerbations of fibrotic hypersensitivity pneumonitis. *Chest.* 2008;134:844-50.

79. Miyazaki Y, Tateishi T, Akashi T, et al. Clinical predictors in histologic appearance of acute exacerbation in chronic hypersensitivity pneumonitis. *Chest.* 2008;134:1265-70.

80. Park IN, Kim DS, Shim TS, et al. Acute exacerbation of interstitial pneumonia other than idiopathic pulmonary fibrosis. *Chest.* 2007;132:214-20.

81. Kondoh Y, Taniguchi H, Kitachi M, et al. Acute exacerbation of interstitial pneumonia following surgical lung biopsy. *Respir Med.* 2006;100:1757-9.

82. Hiwatari N, Shimura S, Takishima T, et al. Bronchoalveolar lavage as a possible cause of acute exacerbation in idiopathic pulmonary fibrosis patients. *Tohoku J Exp Med.* 1994;174:379-86.

83. Honore I, Nunes H, Groussard O, et al. Acute respiratory failure after interferon-gamma therapy of end-stage pulmonary fibrosis. *Am J Respir Crit Care Med.* 2003;167:953-7.

84. Takeda A, Enomoto T, Sanuki N, et al. Acute exacerbation of subclinical idiopathic pulmonary fibrosis triggered by hypofractionated stereotactic body radiotherapy in a patient with primary lung cancer and slightly focal honeycombing. *Radiat Med.* 2008; 26:504-7.

85. Kim DS, Park JH, Park BK, et al. Acute exacerbation of idiopathic pulmonary fibrosis: frequency and clinical features. *Eur Respir J.* 2006;27:143-50.

86. Okamoto T, Ichiyasu H, Ichikado K, et al. Clinical analysis of the acute exacerbation in patients with idiopathic pulmonary fibrosis. *Nihon Kokyuki Gakkai Zasshi.* 2006;44: 359-67.

87. Kubo H, Nakayama K, Yanai M, et al. Anti-coagulant therapy for idiopathic pulmonary fibrosis. *Chest.* 2005;128:1475-82.

88. Azuma A, Nukiwa T, Tsuboi E. Double-blind placebo-controled trial of pirfenidone in patients with idiopathic pulmonary fibrosis. *Am J Respir Crit Care Med.* 2005;171: 1040-4.

89. Akira M, Kozuka T, Yamamoto S, et al. Computer tomography findings in acute exacerbation of idiopathic pulmonary fibrosis. *Am J Respir Crit Care Med.* 2008;178: 372-8.

90. Akira M, Hamada H, Sakatani M, et al. CT findings during the phase of accelerated deterioration in patients with idiopathic pulmonary fibrosis. *Am J Roentgenol.* 1997; 168:79-83.

91. Nakamura M, Ogura T, Miyazawa N, et al. Outcome of patients of acute exacerbations of idiopathic pulmonary fibrosis (IPF) treated with sivelestat and the prognostic value of serum KL-6 and surfactant protein D. *Nihon Kyuki Gakkaie Zasshi.* 2007;45:455-9.

92. Yokoyama A, Kohno N, Hamada H, et al. Circulating KL-6 predicts the outcome of rapidly progressive idiopathic pulmonary fibrosis. *Am J Respir Crit Care Med.* 1998;158: 1680-4.

93. Ishizaka A, Matsuda T, Albertine KH, et al. Elevation of KL-6, a lung epithelial cell marker in plasma and epithelial lining fluid in acute respiratory distress syndrome. *Am J Physiol Lung Cell Mol Physiol.* 2004;286:L1088-94.

94. Eisner MD, Parsons P, Matthay MA, et al. Plasma surfactant protein levels and clinical outcomes in patients with acute lung injury. *Thorax.* 2003;58:983-8.

95. Queisser MA, Kouri FM, Konigshoff, et al. Loss of RAGE in pulmonary fibrosis: molecular relations to functional changes in pulmonary cell types. *Am J Respir Cell Mol Biol.* 2008;39:337-45.

96. Englert JM, Hanford LE, Kaminski N, et al. A role for the receptor for advanced glycation end products in idiopathic pulmonary fibrosis. *Am J Pathol.* 2008;172:583-91.

97. Uchida T, Shirasawa M, Ware LB, et al. Receptor for advanced glycation end-products is a marker of type 1 cell injury and acute lung injury. *Am J Respir Crit Care Med.* 2006; 173:1008-15.

98. Ware LB, Eisner MD, Thompson BT, et al. The significance of von Willebrand factor in septic and non-septic patients with acute lung injury. *Am J Respir Crit Care Med.* 2004; 170:766-72.

99. Collard HR, Calfee CS, Wolters PJ, et al. Plasma biomarker profiles in acute exacerbations of idiopathic pulmonary fibrosis. *Am J Physiol Lung Cell and Mol Physiol.* 2010;299: L3-L7.

100. Ware LB, Matthay ME, Parsons PE, et al. Pathogenetic and prognostic significance of altered coagulation and fibrinolysis in acute lung injury/acute respiratory distress syndrome. *Crit Care Med.* 2007;35:1821-8.

101. Huie TJ, Moss M, Frankel SK. What can biomarkers tell us about the pathogenesis of acute exacerbations of idiopathic pulmonary fibrosis? *Am J Physiol Lung Cell and Mol Physiol.* 2010;299:L1-L2.

102. Ware LB, Koyama T, Billheimer DD, et al. Prognostic and pathogenetic value of combining clinical and biochemical indices in patients with acute lung injury. *Chest.* 2010;137:288-96.

103. Selman M, Pardo A. Roll of epithelial cells in idiopathic pulmonary fibrosis: from innocent targets to serial killers. *Proc Am Thorac Soc.* 2006;3:364-72.

104. Huie TJ, Olson AL, Cosgrove GP, et al. A detailed evaluation of acute respiratory decline in patients with fibrotic lung disease: etiology and outcomes. *Respir.* 2010;15:909-17.

105. Moeller A, Gilpin SE, Ask K, et al. Circulating fibrocytes are an indicator of poor prognosis in idiopathic pulmonary fibrosis. *Am J Respir Crit Care Med.* 2009;179: 588-94.

106. Andersson-Sjoland A, de Alba CG, Nihlberg K, et al. Fibrocytes are a potential source of lung fibroblasts in idiopathic pulmonary fibrosis. *Int J Biochem Cell Biol.* 2008;40: 2129-40.

107. Suga M, Iyonaga K, Okamoto T, et al. Characteristic elevation of matrix metalloproteinase activity in idiopathic interstitial pneumonias. *Am J Respir Crit Care Med.* 2000;162: 1949-56.

108. Yu Q, Stamenkovic I. Cell surface-localized matrix metalloproteinase-9 proteolytically activates TGF-beta and promotes tumor invasion and angiogenesis. *Genes Dev.* 2000; 14:163-76.

109. Gunther A, Mosavi P, Ruppert C, et al. Enhanced tissue factor pathway activity and fibrin turnover in the alveolar compartment of patients with interstitial lung disease. *Thromb Haemost.* 2000;83:853-60.

110. Armanios MY, Chen JJ, Cogan JD, et al. Telomerase mutations in families with idiopathic pulmonary fibrosis. *N Eng J Med.* 2007;356:1317-26.

111. Tsakiri K, Cronkhite JT, Kuan PJ, et al. Adult-onset pulmonary fibrosis caused by mutations in telomerase. *Proc Natl Acad Sci USA.* 2007;104:7552-7.

112. Inase N, Sawada M, Ohtani Y, et al. Cyclosporin A followed by the treatment of acute exacerbation of idiopathic pulmonary fibrosis with corticosteroid. *Intern Med.* 2003;42: 565-70.

113. Sakamoto S, Homma S, Miyamoto A, et al. Cyclosporin A in the treatment of acute exacerbation of idiopathic pulmonary fibrosis. *Intern Med.* 2010;49:109-15.

114. Homma S, Sakamoto S, Kawabata M, et al. Cyclosporin treatment in steroid-resistant and acutely exacerbated interstitial pneumonia. *Intern Med.* 2005;44:1144-50.

115. Taniguchi H, Ebina M, Kondoh Y, et al. Pirfenidone in idiopathic pulmonary fibrosis. *Eur Respir J.* 2010;35:821-9.

116. Song JW, Hong SB, Lian CM, et al. Acute exacerbations of idiopathic pulmonary fibrosis: incidence, risk factors, and outcome. *Eur Respir J.* 2011;37:356-63. Epub July 2010.

117. Saydain G, Islam A, Affesa B, et al. Outcome of patients with idiopathic pulmonary fibrosis admitted to the intensive care unit. *Am J Respir Crit Care Med.* 2002;166: 839-42.

118. Blivet S, Philit F, Sab JM, et al. Outcome of patients with idiopathic pulmonary fibrosis admitted to the ICU for respiratory failure. *Chest.* 2001;120:209-12.

119. Mallick S. Outcome of patients with idiopathic pulmonary fibrosis (IPF) ventilated in intensive care unit. *Respir Med.* 2008;102:1355-9.

120. Rangappa P, Moran JL. Outcome of patients admitted to the intensive care unit with idiopathic pulmonary fibrosis. *Crit Care Resusc.* 2009;11:102-9.

CHAPTER 6

Acute Pulmonary Exacerbations of Sarcoidosis

Efstratios Panselinas,
Vlassis Polychronopoulos, Marc A Judson

INTRODUCTION

Sarcoidosis is a disease of unknown cause which is characterized by the presence of noncaseating granulomas in many organs. The immune process that causes the granulomatous inflammation of sarcoidosis is not well understood. However, it is believed that the immunopathogenesis begins with antigen engulfment and subsequent processing by antigen presenting cells (APC) followed by the presentation of processed antigen to T cell receptors via HLA class II molecules. This results in the production of cytokines of the T-helper 1 class leading to T cell proliferation, monocyte recruitment, and finally, granuloma formation.[1] The putative antigen(s) responsible for these events is presently unknown. Although sarcoidosis can affect any organ, pulmonary involvement is most common. Abnormalities on chest radiographs are detected in 85–95% of patients.[2] Cough, dyspnea, and chest pain are typical presenting symptoms; however, 30–60% of patients are asymptomatic at presentation and their disease is detected on the basis of abnormal radiographic findings.[3-5]

Patients may develop acute pulmonary exacerbations of sarcoidosis (APES).[6-9] APES may be problematic to be differentiated from other pulmonary illnesses. Although corticosteroids are considered as the treatment of choice for pulmonary sarcoidosis, the precise corticosteroid dose recommendations for APES have not been established. In this chapter, we focus on the definition, pathophysiology, diagnosis, and treatment of APES.

DEFINITION

There is no consensus definition for APES, in contrast to exacerbations of other pulmonary diseases (i.e., chronic obstructive pulmonary disease (COPD), idiopathic pulmonary fibrosis (IPF)). Gottlieb and colleagues defined sarcoidosis relapses as recurrences of the clinical manifestations of disease severe enough to warrant treatment, following at least one month of a remission of symptoms without administration of corticosteroids.[8] These authors did not focus exclusively on pulmonary exacerbations. Two other recent clinical studies defined APES as new or worsening pulmonary symptoms in patients with known sarcoidosis, combined with ≥ 10% decrease of forced vital capacity (FVC) or forced expiratory volume in 1 second (FEV_1) from baseline that cannot be attributed to another cause (i.e., infection).[6-10] The ultimate diagnosis of APES also requires a response to antisarcoidosis medications, usually in the form of corticosteroids. However, a patient with possible APES may be experiencing an exacerbation of an alternative pulmonary disease such as asthma or COPD. Therefore, such alternate conditions should be carefully excluded before a diagnosis of APES is established.[10]

We suggest that APES should be defined as the recurrence or deterioration of pulmonary symptoms that cannot be explained by another cause, combined with a decline in spirometry (≥ 10% decrease from previous baseline FVC with or without FEV_1). The decline should occur within 3 months from the onset of symptoms.

EPIDEMIOLOGY

The frequency of APES in patients with sarcoidosis is 14–75%.[8,9,11-14] The wide variation is likely the result of differences in study populations, dose and duration of corticosteroid treatment, and length of follow-up. In addition, the definition of APES is variable between studies, as the majority of them do not focus exclusively in pulmonary exacerbations. Relapses of pulmonary disease have been described in patients with or without treatment. In a large observational study from the United States, the rate of sarcoidosis relapse was 74%.[8] Although the authors included patients with extrapulmonary sarcoidosis relapses, 51 out of 86 patients (59%) had a pulmonary exacerbation of the disease. In European study with a predominantly white population, relapses of sarcoidosis occurred in 37% of patients with half of them affecting the lung.[12]

There are minimal data concerning the demographics of APES. Most demographic associations with relapses of sarcoidosis do not specifically address pulmonary exacerbations, but rather exacerbations of sarcoidosis in general. Therefore, the demographics of APES must, in part, be extrapolated from these studies. African Americans are thought to be at higher risk of exacerbations than Caucasians.[14] African Americans of both genders and Caucasian women appear to be at higher risk of exacerbations as compared to Caucasian men.[8]

Certain clinical presentations of sarcoidosis are associated with an increased probability of relapse, whereas other presentations are relatively protective of relapse. Patients with erythema nodosum and bilateral hilar adenopathy usually have spontaneous remission of sarcoidosis without recurrence, although such patients may suffer relapses.[15] Patients who present with musculoskeletal symptoms also seem to have a greater likelihood of relapse.[8]

Treatment with corticosteroids has been implicated as a risk factor for exacerbations when corticosteroids are withdrawn.[8] Gottlieb and coworkers demonstrated that patients with corticosteroid induced remissions had a relapse rate of 74% as compared to only 8% in the group with spontaneous remissions. In addition, a higher corticosteroid dose has been described as risk factor for relapse.[12] Rizzato and colleagues retrospectively reviewed the outcome of sarcoidosis patients who had corticosteroids tapered after a corticosteroid induced remission. Patients who relapsed had received a higher corticosteroid dose (median dose 17 mg/d) as compared to those who did not experience an exacerbation (median dose 10.6 mg/d). In contradistinction to these two reports, a study of 172 United States sarcoidosis patients with predominantly white population showed that treatment with corticosteroids was associated with a lower rate of relapse (22%) as compared to that of the previous studies.[16] These studies suggest that corticosteroid therapy is a risk factor for exacerbations, although demographic factors and the severity of disease also affect risk. These data also highlight the danger of the indiscriminate use of corticosteroids for the treatment of sarcoidosis. A significant percentage of sarcoidosis patients will undergo spontaneous remission. The unnecessary use of corticosteroids in sarcoidosis patients with a high likelihood of spontaneous remission not only exposes them to the risk of corticosteroid side effects but may also increase the risk of relapse.

Interferon (INF) treatment for hepatitis[17] appears to be a risk factor for exacerbations of sarcoidosis. This is understandable because INF-gamma is an integral cytokine involved in the formation of the sarcoid granuloma.[18] Treatment with INF-alfa and INF-beta has been reported to cause a sarcoid-like syndrome in patients without previous sarcoidosis.[19] We suspect that activation of granulomatous inflammation in sarcoidosis may depend not only on the drugs effect upon the immune system but also on whether the putative sarcoidosis antigen has previously been cleared.[20]

Highly active antiretroviral therapy (HAART) for the acquired immunodeficiency syndrome (AIDS) has been implicated as a risk factor for development or recurrence of sarcoidosis.[21] Human immunodeficiency virus (HIV) infection results in destruction of CD4+ T cells which are required for the formation of granulomas. HAART therapy results in reconstitution of immunity, specifically by increasing CD4+ T cells that may heighten the granulomatous response to the sarcoid antigen (*vide infra*).

Table 6-1 enlists the demographics, clinical sarcoidosis presentations, and risk factors associated with APES.

PATHOGENESIS OF APES

The immunopathogenesis of the sarcoidosis has been characterized in three phases.[22] During the initial phase, an unknown antigen is engulfed by antigen

Table 6-1	Risk Factors for APES	
Demographic factors	**Treatment**	
African Americans	Corticosteroid induced remission,	
Caucasian women	especially with moderate to high doses of corticosteroids	
Presentation		
Dyspnea during initial presentation of sarcoidosis	**Other factors**	
	Interferon treatment for other diseases	
Previous bouts of APES	Highly active antiretroviral therapy in HIV patients	

presenting cells, processed and presented to CD4+ T cells via HLA class II molecules. Subsequently, T cells of the Th1 class are activated. It is thought that a genetic predisposition to the development of sarcoidosis depends at least in part on the individual's specific HLA genotype. In the second phase, the ongoing presentation of the antigen to Th1 cells results in the production of Th1-related cytokines that drive the formation of granuloma through the local proliferation of T-lymphocytes and recruitment of monocytes. The third phase involves the clearance of the antigen causing downregulation of the immune response and spontaneous resolution of the granulomatous inflammation. A shift in Th1/Th2 response with an effective humoral response and clearance of the immunocomplexes has been implicated as the mechanism of antigen clearance.[23]

In some sarcoidosis patients, ongoing granulomatous inflammation is observed that results in chronic disease. It seems plausible that during APES, the antigen that caused the granulomatous inflammation of sarcoidosis was not effectively cleared and caused an exacerbation of the disease when antisarcoidosis therapy was withdrawn. This schema is supported by the fact that treatment of sarcoidosis with corticosteroids, methotrexate, or infliximab attenuates the granulomatous inflammation and improves symptoms but does not alter the natural course of the disease.[16,24-27] These therapies probably prevent clearance of the presumed antigen, allowing the disease to relapse when therapy is withdrawn. In addition, exacerbations of sarcoidosis have been described in HIV infected patients after institution of HAART.[21] It is possible that the putative antigen is present in those patients but their low CD4+ count prior to HAART precludes the development of an effective granulomatous immune response. After HAART is initiated, the resultant increase in CD4+ lymphocytes causes an immune response similar to the immune reconstitution inflammatory initial syndrome seen in tuberculosis, resulting in granulomatous inflammation and an exacerbation of the disease.

Recurrence after spontaneous remission of sarcoidosis has been described.[15] In these cases, complete clearance of the responsible antigen followed by re-exposure to the same or a different antigen has been suggested as the mechanism of the exacerbation.

DIAGNOSIS OF APES

APES may occur in patients receiving antisarcoidosis medication or in patients who are not receiving any therapy. In one series of 36 cases of APES, 28 (78%) developed the condition while receiving less than or equal to 5 mg of daily prednisone equivalent. No patient developed APES who was receiving more than 10 mg of daily prednisone.[6] When APES occurs after sarcoidosis treatment is discontinued, it usually develops within one year; however, 20% of relapses occur more than 1 year after cessation of therapy and 10% occur after two or more years.[8] In patients with chronic stable disease, exacerbations usually, occur when the daily corticosteroid dose is tapered below 15 mg of prednisone equivalent.[6,14]

Patients with APES present with new or increasing dyspnea, cough, wheezing, or chest pain. In some patients, nonspecific symptoms such as fever, night sweats, or fatigue may predominate. APES can occur in patients who only had extrapulmonary manifestations of sarcoidosis previously.[8] There are no physical examination findings specific for APES. Static lung volumes and diffusing capacity measurements have not been examined during APES. Cardiopulmonary exercise testing and 6-minute walk testing (6-MWT) are more sensitive for the detection of changes in exercise performance in patients with stable disease but are cumbersome to use, and their sensitivity and specificity for the diagnosis of APES is unknown.

The role of the chest radiograph (CXR) in the diagnosis of APES is controversial. Radiographic abnormalities correlate with symptoms and PFTs during the course of the disease.[28,29] However, in a recent study, the use of International Labor Organization profusion score in CXR was not a reliable test to detect a pulmonary exacerbation of the disease.[10] Interestingly, majority of chest radiographs of patients with APES demonstrated improvement (19%) or no change (32%) in profusion score. An explanation for these findings is that it is problematic to detect new parenchymal lung opacities associated with APES in sarcoidosis patients with significant parenchymal opacities at baseline. In addition, parenchymal sarcoidosis has a predilection for the bronchovascular bundles and subpleural areas, and it is relatively problematic to discern abnormalities on the chest radiograph in these areas. However, a CXR is still recommended for presumed APES not to establish the diagnosis but to exclude alternative diagnoses that could explain the clinical findings. Chest computed tomography (CT) scanning is superior to chest radiographs in delineating parenchymal abnormalities in sarcoidosis, but it has not been evaluated during APES.

Biological markers have been used for detecting disease activity. Serum angiotensin converting enzyme (ACE) is elevated in 30–80% of patients with sarcoidosis and may be a marker of granulomatous burden.[3] An increase in serum ACE levels may indicate APES when associated with typical clinical features and reductions in pulmonary function.[30] Corticosteroids lead to a reduction in the serum

ACE level.[31] Therefore, a subsequent increase after corticosteroids withdrawal may represent persistent disease activity and not clinical worsening.[32] An elevation of serum ACE in isolation, without any other clinical stigmata of APES is insufficient to escalate treatment.[7] Other biomarkers of disease activity such as soluble IL-2R have been suggested as potential surrogates for disease progression.[33,34] However, no such marker has been studied during APES, so that their measurement cannot be routinely recommended.

Bronchoalveolar lavage (BAL) with examination of lymphocytes subpopulations has been used to gauge disease activity of sarcoidosis.[35] In addition, BAL may be helpful in excluding alternative causes of pulmonary decompensation other than APES such as infections. Although BAL should usually discriminate APES from alternative diagnoses, we believe that the diagnosis of APES can usually be made on clinical grounds, without the need for this invasive procedure. BAL should be reserved for atypical presentations or when a patient with presumed APES fails to respond rapidly to therapy (within two weeks).

In the case of a patient with pulmonary sarcoidosis who is present with symptoms and signs suggestive of APES, spirometry should be performed in order to confirm the decline in FVC or FEV_1. As mentioned previously, a CXR should be routinely performed not to confirm APES but rather to exclude alternative diagnoses. Additional testing may be required if certain specific alternative diagnoses are considered, such as a complete blood count and sputum cultures when the presentation is suggestive of pulmonary infection.

Table 6-2 enlists the major alternative diagnostic considerations when APES is considered. Pulmonary infections, such as acute bronchitis and pneumonia, are common in sarcoidosis patients who often require immunosuppressive medications.[36] Concern for infection should be especially heightened in potential APES patients receiving baseline highly immunosuppressive medications such as high-dose corticosteroids or infliximab. Symptoms which would raise the suspicion of lung infection in a patient with possible APES would include a cough productive of purulent sputum, fever, night sweats, significant weight loss, and hemoptysis. However, all of these symptoms may be found with APES, although they are not typical. An elevated white blood cell count with the presence of immature forms may also suggest infection as an alternative diagnosis to APES. A CXR that reveals a localized alveolar opacity strongly favors a diagnosis of infection rather than APES. When APES and pulmonary infection cannot be clearly distinguished, one approach would be to empirically treat the patient with antibiotics and monitor the patient for improvement. If the patient fails to improve, such a patient could then be treated for APES. An alternative approach in this situation would be to perform more expensive with or without invasive testing such as chest CT scanning and bronchoscopy with BAL.

Table 6-2 Differential Diagnosis of APES

	APES	Pneumonia	Bronchitis	Tuberculosis	Asthma	Congestive heart failure	Pulmonary hypertension
History	History of sarcoidosis Previous APES Receiving ≤ 10 mg prednisone daily equivalent	Risk factors for pneumonia (e.g., immunosuppression, aspiration)	History of smoking History of previous bronchitis	Risk of tuberculosis exposure History of positive tuberculin skin test	History of asthma Exposure to asthma triggers (pollen, viral infections, etc.)	History of congestive heart failure History compatible with fluid overload	Dyspnea failing to respond to corticosteroids, bronchodilators, or antibiotics
Symptoms (relative frequency)							
Dyspnea	+4	+2	+1	+1	+4	+4	+4
Orthopnea	0	0	0	0	0	+4	0
Cough	+4	+4	+4	+4	+4	+2	+1
Sputum	+2	+3	+3	+4	+1	+1	0
Wheezing	+3	+1	+3	0	+4	+1	0
Chest pain	+2	+2	0	0	+3	+3	+2
Night sweats	+1	+2	0	+3	0	0	0
Fever	+1	+4	+1	+4	+1	0	0
Rigors	0	+3	0	0	0	0	0
Weight loss	+1	0	0	+3	0	0	0
Peripheral edema	0	0	0	0	0	+3	+2

Continued

Continued

	APES	Pneumonia	Bronchitis	Tuberculosis	Asthma	Congestive heart failure	Pulmonary hypertension
Physical findings	Normal, occasionally wheezing	Fever, focal signs of pulmonary consolidation	Focal or diffuse rhonchi/wheezing	Normal/focal or diffuse rhonchi	Diffuse polyphonic wheezing	Peripheral edema ↑JVP S3/S4 on cardiac examination Diffuse crackles/rhonchi	Accentuated P2 ↑JVP Right ventricular heave Peripheral edema
Laboratory tests	Spirometry: Decline of FVC and/or FEV$_1$ CXR: New or worsening parenchymal infiltrates, new or worsening parenchymal nodules, no change in CXR is common	↑WBC CXR: Consolidation	↑WBC CXR: No changes	TST: + CXR: Cavities/ focal alveolar opacities/ pleural reaction HRCT: Cavities/tree in bud pattern Sputum/BAL: Stains with or without cultures + for mycobacteria Histology: Necrotic granulomas	Spirometry: Obstruction on spirometry with a bronchodilator response CXR: Normal or hyperinflation	ECG: Signs of LV hypertrophy, ischemic heart disease or rhythm disturbance Echo: ↓ EF, diastolic dysfunction CXR: Central alveolar opacities, pleural effusions ↑BNP	ECG: signs of RV hypertrophy PFTs: ↓ DLCO with relatively preserved spirometry ↑BNP Echo: ↑RVSP, signs of RV failure RHC: mPAP > 25 mmHg and Pcwp ≤ 15 mmHg

RVSP, right ventricular systolic pressure; RHC, right heart catheterization; mPAP, mean pulmonary artery pressure; Pcwp, pulmonary capillary wedge pressure; BNP, brain natriuretic peptide; TST, tuberculin skin test; ↑, elevated; ↓, reduced; +, positive test 0 (almost never) to +4 (almost always).

Active pulmonary tuberculosis may be particularly problematic to differentiate from APES. As previously mentioned, both conditions may be associated with a productive cough, fever, night sweats, and weight loss. Tuberculosis is more likely to result in lung cavitation and cause pleural reaction. Chest CT scans may help differentiate these two entities, as sarcoidosis is typically associated with parenchymal disease along the bronchovascular bundle, while tuberculosis typically reveals lung cavitation and endobronchial spread of disease. The granulomas of sarcoidosis tend to be non-necrotic while those of tuberculosis are usually necrotic. However, both the conditions can display necrotic and non-necrotic granulomatous inflammation. Obviously, stains and cultures for mycobacteria are essential in making this differentiation. In problematic cases, it may be appropriate to treat first for tuberculosis and then for sarcoidosis or to administer therapy for both diseases concomitantly if the patient is gravely ill. In these cases, it is essential to obtain adequate stains and cultures for mycobacteria before initiating antituberculosis therapy.

Cardiogenic pulmonary edema should also be considered in patients with sarcoidosis and pulmonary symptoms. Pulmonary edema could be a complication of cardiac sarcoidosis or more likely, heart disease related to diabetes or hypertension from chronic corticosteroid use. If signs or symptoms of congestive heart failure are present such as typical angina, orthopnea, or peripheral edema, then an electrocardiograph, echocardiogram with or without serum B-type natriuretic peptide (BNP) levels may be useful to differentiate APES from pulmonary edema. A CXR may also be of value in this instance.

Pulmonary hypertension is a potential complication of sarcoidosis,[37-39] and it needs to be considered when evaluating a patient for APES. Patients with sarcoidosis-associated pulmonary hypertension (SAPH) are usually present with dyspnea on exertion.[40] Physical examination may reveal an accentuated P2 and in advance cases, signs of right heart failure such as right ventricular heave, elevated jugular pressure, and lower extremity edema. These patients often have resting hypoxemia. The dyspnea from SAPH is usually not reflected by spirometry which is often within the normal range. This discordance between spirometry and dyspnea is a clue to the diagnosis of SAPH and assists in distinguishing this diagnosis from APES. Similarly, spirometry and diffusing capacity are typically discordant in SAPH, usually with the former relatively normal and the latter usually quite reduced. This is another clue to the diagnosis of SAPH. SAPH patients usually have a diminished 6-minute-walk distance and demonstrate significant oxygen desaturation that is usually more severe than with APES. All these pulmonary function test findings may be used as screening tools for SAPH. When these tests suggest SAPH as a potential diagnosis, an echocardiogram should be performed with the estimation of right ventricular systolic pressure. It should be noted that if the estimated right ventricular systolic pressure is normal or cannot be estimated on echocardiography, SAPH cannot be excluded.[41] Echocardiography may also be useful to exclude left ventricular dysfunction. If there is a high index of suspicion of SAPH or if echocardiography suggests pulmonary hypertension, right heart catheterization is mandatory to confirm the diagnosis and the exclusion of left ventricular dysfunction which can contribute to the elevated pulmonary pressures.

Finally, exacerbations of asthma and COPD should be excluded before the diagnosis of APES can be secured. This is highly problematic because these diseases share common symptoms and physical findings with APES. In addition, like APES, these diseases respond to corticosteroid therapy.

Patients with asthma exacerbations usually have a prior history of asthma and often a family history of asthma. A search should be made for asthma triggers such as pollens, environmental exposures, and viral infections. Wheezing cough, dyspnea, and chest tightness are the prominent symptoms, which unfortunately are not dissimilar from APES. It is underappreciated that pulmonary sarcoidosis often results in wheezing and airflow obstruction from endobronchial disease or airway distortion related to sarcoidosis associated fibrosis. One potentially differentiating feature is that asthmatics usually respond to bronchodilator therapy whereas APES patients uncommonly do. On many occasions, it may be impossible to differentiate asthma from APES. Fortunately, both conditions respond to corticosteroid therapy although APES has a higher rate of relapse and this may be an eventual clue to the diagnosis.

COPD is characterized by chronic airflow limitation. Cigarette smoking is the main etiological factor. Cigarette smoking history is protective of sarcoidosis,[42] and so this distinction is often not problematic. Exacerbations of COPD are present with increasing dyspnea, sputum production, and changes in sputum purulence. Again, all of these symptoms may be present with APES. Bacterial and viral infections are responsible for the majority of COPD exacerbations. Bronchodilators are the mainstay of treatment along with the antibiotics and corticosteroids. The differentiation between APES and a COPD exacerbation in a smoking patient with sarcoidosis is impossible, and both the conditions should then be treated concomitantly. Spirometry is generally not useful to identify the disease process, as both APES and COPD may show worsening airflow obstruction.

Treatment

APES should be treated in order to ameliorate symptoms and potentially prevent the development of fibrosis from ongoing granulomatous inflammation. An approach to treatment of APES is shown in figure 6-1. The medications that can be used are shown in table 6-3.

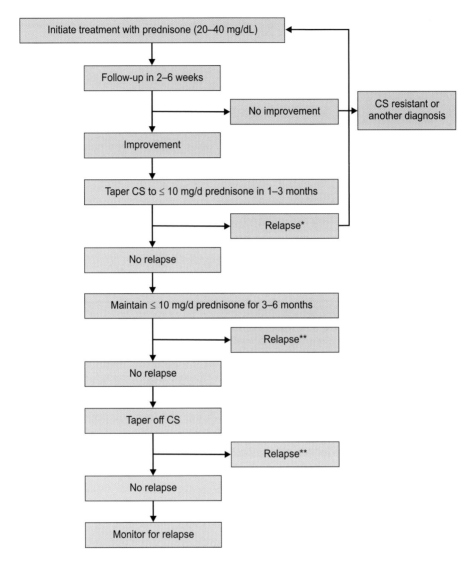

Figure 6-1 Treatment algorithm for APES. *Consider corticosteroid sparing agents if the prednisone dose cannot be maintained at ≤ 10 mg/d; **Attempt to maintain the lowest effective corticosteroid dose. The decision to add corticosteroid sparing agents should be individualized. CS, corticosteroids.

Corticosteroids are the treatment of choice for APES. The suggested initial corticosteroid dose is 20-40 mg of daily prednisone equivalent.[7,8,12] A small retrospective study of APES suggested that 20 mg of prednisone for three weeks is sufficient for the improvement of symptoms and return of pulmonary function to

Table 6-3	Reported Medications for Treatment of APES	
Medication	Dose	Indication
Prednisone	20–40 mg/d	Initial treatment
Methotrexate	10–25 mg/wk	Corticosteroid sparing agent
Chloroquine	250–750 mg/d	Corticosteroid sparing agent
Infliximab	3–5 mg/kg initially, week 2, then every 4–8 weeks	Steroid sparing agent. May be used as initial treatment in patients with corticosteroid resistant sarcoidosis who suffer with an APES

the baseline.[6] This study only addressed the initial acute treatment of APES and not the method for tapering the corticosteroid dose. Failure to improve during the first month of corticosteroid treatment suggests the rare possibility that the APES is corticosteroid resistant or, more likely, that there is an alternative cause responsible for the pulmonary dysfunction.[43]

Follow-up is recommended 2–6 weeks after the initial treatment of APES. Corticosteroids should be tapered when pulmonary symptoms and function return near baseline. Tapering to a maintenance dose of ≤ 10 mg of prednisone is usually completed in 1–3 months. The duration of maintenance phase is not clearly defined and should be individualized dependent upon the patient's response. In general, an attempt should be made to discontinue corticosteroids in 3–9 months. This may depend upon many factors including the corticosteroid dose at the time of the exacerbation, a history of corticosteroid dependence, the frequency of previous bouts of APES, and whether the patient has experienced or is at high risk for corticosteroid side effects. The time until discontinuation may be extended for years or the therapy may need to be lifelong if the patient has failed previous corticosteroid tapers. The corticosteroid dose should not be routinely tapered more rapidly than every two weeks, since this is usually the minimal amount of time for a clinical relapse to occur if anti-inflammatory therapy is inadequate.[7] Patients with APES, who are treated and successfully tapered off corticosteroids, require continued monitoring. Although it has been recommended that patients should be monitored for one year after completion of corticosteroid therapy,[44] 20% of sarcoidosis relapses occur one year after cessation of corticosteroid therapy and 10% occur beyond two years.[8] We, therefore, recommend that monitoring should be continued for a minimum of two years after an episode of APES. When corticosteroids cannot be successfully tapered off, the lowest effective maintenance dose should be used. Although corticosteroid dosing should be individualized based on the risk of potential side effects and previous episodes of APES, it has been suggested that if the daily maintenance corticosteroid dose cannot be lowered to ≤ 10 mg of prednisone equivalent, the corticosteroid taper has not been successful and a corticosteroid sparing agent should be added.[45]

Methotrexate has been used as a corticosteroid sparing agent for both acute and chronic sarcoidosis.[25,46] Methotrexate cannot be advocated initially for APES because the drug usually requires 1-9 months of use to be effective.[47] Methotrexate is most commonly used in conjunction with corticosteroids as a corticosteroid sparing agent in order to reduce the potential toxicity of corticosteroids. Methotrexate may cause liver toxicity or bone marrow suppression. Therefore, monitoring of serum transaminases and complete blood counts is required. Liver biopsy has been recommended after a cumulative methotrexate dose of 1-1.5 g.[48]

The antimalarial chloroquine has been shown to reduce the rate of relapse of chronic pulmonary sarcoidosis.[49] Chloroquine has a significant potential of causing retinal toxicity, and therefore, requires ophthalmologic examinations every 6-12 months.[50] As the maximum benefit from chloroquine requires six months of treatment, it cannot be solely used as the initial agent for APES. Other agents such as azathioprine and pentoxifylline have been shown to have corticosteroid sparing effects in a small number of patients.[51-53] Their role in APES has not been examined.

Thalidomide has been tested as a steroid sparing agent in patients receiving corticosteroids and having a history of APES within the previous two years.[54] While receiving this drug, a minority of patients (3 out of 10) were able to reduce their corticosteroid dose without suffering an exacerbation. However, 2 of 10 patients developed APES during the study before tapering the corticosteroid dose and a majority (9 out of 10) had to reduce the thalidomide dose because of intolerable side effects. These data suggest that thalidomide is not a very reliable agent to protect against APES.

Infliximab is a chimeric monoclonal antibody against TNF-alfa which has been shown to be effective in refractory sarcoidosis. Two double-blind, randomized, placebo-controlled trials showed benefit for infliximab for chronic pulmonary sarcoidosis.[55,56] The drug is typically given intravenously three times within the first six weeks of therapy and then every 4-8 weeks. A beneficial effect of this drug is usually apparent within six weeks of initiating therapy. The rapid response to this agent makes it a consideration for patients with APES who are refractory to CS or cannot be successfully tapered. However, infliximab is highly immunosuppressive and is associated with opportunistic infections and possibly malignancy, it is also cumbersome to use as it requires intravenous infusion. Finally, the drug is highly costly. For all these reasons, infliximab is not recommended as a routine therapy for APES.

PROGNOSIS

The prognosis of APES is not clearly defined. Three quarters of pulmonary sarcoidosis patients who require therapy will develop APES when corticosteroids are withdrawn. One quarter of patients experience one episode, while half may have multiple bouts of APES.[14] Patients on systemic therapy at the initial presentation, have a more than three fold chance compared to untreated patients to be on treatment after 18-24 months. In addition, the presence of dyspnea at the initial evaluation is predictive of continuous treatment two years later.[57] It is important to be cognizant of these prognostic factors as patients with a high chance of relapse should probably be more closely monitored during treatment withdrawal.

CASE STUDY

A 40-year-old African-American woman sought medical attention for a productive cough of one month's duration. Concomitantly, she had developed dyspnea on ambulation and nocturnal wheezing. She had night sweats, but denied fevers. She had been given a course of quinolone antibiotics by her local physician at the onset of her symptoms with only a transient benefit.

She had a history of sarcoidosis on the basis of a positive Kveim skin test. She had pulmonary sarcoidosis on the basis of hilar lymphadenopathy and diffuse infiltrates on a chest radiograph and liver sarcoidosis on the basis of an elevated serum alkaline phosphatase. Her only medication was prednisone 5 mg daily. She was a lifelong nonsmoker and had no history of tuberculosis or tuberculosis exposure.

Physical examination revealed normal vital signs as well as a normal chest and cardiac examination. She had no peripheral edema. A chest radiograph showed unchanged bilateral hilar adenopathy and diffuse interstitial infiltrates. Although spirometry was in the normal range (FVC of 2.82 liters, 99% of predicted; FEV_1 of 2.23, 94% predicted), there had been a 330 cc decline in FVC and 300 cc decline in FEV_1 compared to four months earlier.

She was presumed to have developed APES and was treated with 20 mg daily of prednisone. She returned two weeks later with complete resolution of her pulmonary symptoms. Spirometry was repeated at that time and had returned to her baseline levels.

Comment on Case

This patient received a clinical diagnosis of APES based on the development of pulmonary symptoms, a decline in spirometry of greater than 10% from baseline and exclusion of alternative causes for this presentation. Pneumonia and bronchitis were reasonable initial considerations. However, her failure to respond to antibiotics, lack of chest radiograph change from baseline, and one month duration of her illness made these possibilities unlikely. The majority of patients who developed APES are receiving 5 mg or less of prednisone daily equivalent.[6] The fact that the chest radiograph remained unchanged is typical of APES, as worsening in radiographic infiltrates occurs in a minority of cases.[10] Corticosteroid therapy usually works rapidly in APES, with resolution of symptoms and spirometric defects occurring within three weeks.[6]

CONCLUSION

Acute pulmonary exacerbations of sarcoidosis commonly occur during the course of pulmonary sarcoidosis. Previous corticosteroid therapy, previous episodes of APES, and African American race are the main risk factors for APES. Patients may present with new or worsening pulmonary symptoms and a decline in pulmonary function. CXR findings in APES are inconsistent, although a CXR is imperative to exclude potential alternative causes. Careful exclusion of other potential causes of pulmonary decompensation is required before the diagnosis of APES can be secured. Corticosteroids are the treatment of choice for APES. Corticosteroid sparing agents should be considered in corticosteroid refractory cases, when high doses of corticosteroids are required, or in patients with a history of previous APES.

REFERENCES

1. Hunninghake GW, Costabel U, Ando M, et al. ATS/ERS/WASOG statement on sarcoidosis. American Thoracic Society/European Respiratory Society/World Association of Sarcoidosis and other Granulomatous Disorders. *Sarcoidosis Vasc Diffuse Lung Dis.* 1999;16:149-73.
2. Mihailovic-Vucinic V, Jovanovic D. Pulmonary sarcoidosis. *Clin Chest Med.* 2008;29: 459-73, viii-ix.
3. Lynch JP, Kazerooni EA, Gay SE. Pulmonary sarcoidosis. *Clin Chest Med.* 1997;18:755-85.
4. Reich JM, Johnson RE. Course and prognosis of sarcoidosis in a nonreferral setting. Analysis of 86 patients observed for 10 years. *Am J Med.* 1985;78:61-7.
5. Hillerdal G, Nou E, Osterman K, et al. Sarcoidosis: epidemiology and prognosis. A 15-year European study. *Am Rev Respir Dis.* 1984;130:29-32.
6. McKinzie BP, Bullington WM, Mazur JE, et al. Efficacy of short-course, low-dose corticosteroid therapy for acute pulmonary sarcoidosis exacerbations. *Am J Med Sci.* 2010;339:1-4.
7. Judson MA. An approach to the treatment of pulmonary sarcoidosis with corticosteroids: the six phases of treatment. *Chest.* 1999;115:1158-65.
8. Gottlieb JE, Israel HL, Steiner RM, et al. Outcome in sarcoidosis. The relationship of relapse to corticosteroid therapy. *Chest.* 1997;111:623-31.
9. Takada K, Ina Y, Noda M, et al. The clinical course and prognosis of patients with severe, moderate, or mild sarcoidosis. *J Clin Epidemiol.* 1993;46:359-66.
10. Judson MA, Gilbert GE, Rodgers JK, et al. The utility of the chest radiograph in diagnosing exacerbations of pulmonary sarcoidosis. *Respirology.* 2008;13:97-102.
11. Nagai S, Handa T, Ito Y, et al. Outcome of sarcoidosis. *Clin Chest Med.* 2008;29:565-74, x.
12. Rizzato G, Montemurro L, Colombo P. The late follow-up of chronic sarcoid patients previously treated with corticosteroids. *Sarcoidosis Vasc Diffuse Lung Dis.* 1998;15:52-8.
13. Hunninghake GW, Gilbert S, Pueringer R, et al. Outcome of the treatment for sarcoidosis. *Am J Respir Crit Care Med.* 1994;149:893-8.
14. Johns CJ, Schonfeld SA, Scott PP, et al. Longitudinal study of chronic sarcoidosis with low-dose maintenance corticosteroid therapy. Outcome and complications. *Ann NY Acad Sci.* 1986;465:702-12.

15. Mana J, Montero A, Vidal M, et al. Recurrent sarcoidosis: a study of 17 patients with 24 episodes of recurrence. *Sarcoidosis Vasc Diffuse Lung Dis.* 2003;20:212-21.

16. Eule H, Weinecke A, Roth I, et al. The possible influence of corticosteroid therapy on the natural course of pulmonary sarcoidosis. Late results of a continuing clinical study. *Ann NY Acad Sci.* 1986;465:695-701.

17. Li SD, Yong S, Srinivas D, et al. Reactivation of sarcoidosis during interferon therapy. *J Gastroenterol.* 2002;37:50-4.

18. Iannuzzi MC, Rybicki BA, Teirstein AS. Sarcoidosis. *N Engl J Med.* 2007;357:2153-65.

19. Alazemi S, Campos MA. Interferon-induced sarcoidosis. *Int J Clin Pract.* 2006;60:201-11.

20. Charlier C, Nunes H, Trinchet JC, et al. Evolution of previous sarcoidosis under type 1 interferons given for severe associated disease. *Eur Respir J.* 2005;25:570-3.

21. Lenner R, Bregman Z, Teirstein AS, et al. Recurrent pulmonary sarcoidosis in HIV infected patients receiving highly active antiretroviral therapy. *Chest.* 2001;119:978-81.

22. Grutters JC, Drent M, JMM. Sarcoidosis. *Interstitial Lung Dis.* 2009;126-54.

23. Moller DR, Chen ES. Genetic basis of remitting sarcoidosis: triumph of the trimolecular complex? *Am J Respir Cell Mol Biol.* 2002;27:391-5.

24. Panselinas E, Rodgers JK, Judson MA. Clinical outcomes in sarcoidosis after cessation of infliximab treatment. *Respirology.* 2009;14:522-8.

25. Lower EE, Baughman RP. Prolonged use of methotrexate for sarcoidosis. *Arch Intern Med.* 1995;155:846-51.

26. Zaki MH, Lyons HA, Leilop L, et al. Corticosteroid therapy in sarcoidosis. A five-year, controlled follow-up study. *NY State J Med.* 1987;87:496-9.

27. Israel HL, Fouts DW, Beggs RA. A controlled trial of prednisone treatment of sarcoidosis. *Am Rev Respir Dis.* 1973;107:609-14.

28. Muers MF, Middleton WG, Gibson GJ, et al. A simple radiographic scoring method for monitoring pulmonary sarcoidosis: relations between radiographic scores, dyspnoea grade and respiratory function in the British Thoracic Society Study of Long-Term Corticosteroid Treatment. *Sarcoidosis Vasc Diffuse Lung Dis.* 1997;14:46-56.

29. McLoud TC, Epler GR, Gaensler EA, et al. A radiographic classification for sarcoidosis: physiologic correlation. *Invest Radiol.* 1982;17:129-38.

30. Lieberman J, Schleissner LA, Nosal A, et al. Clinical correlations of serum angiotensin-converting enzyme (ACE) in sarcoidosis. A longitudinal study of serum ACE, 67 gallium scans, chest roentgenograms, and pulmonary function. *Chest.* 1983;84:522-8.

31. Ainslie GM, Benatar SR. Serum angiotensin converting enzyme in sarcoidosis: sensitivity and specificity in diagnosis: correlations with disease activity, duration, extra-thoracic involvement, radiographic type and therapy. *Q J Med.* 1985;55:253-70.

32. Gronhagen-Riska C, Selroos O, Niemisto M. Angiotensin converting enzyme. V. Serum levels as monitors of disease activity in corticosteroid-treated sarcoidosis. *Eur J Respir Dis.* 1980;61:113-22.

33. Ziegenhagen MW, Benner UK, et al. Sarcoidosis: TNF-alfa release from alveolar macro-phages and serum level of sIL-2R are prognostic markers. *Am J Respir Crit Care Med.* 1997;156:1586-92.

34. Grutters JC, Fellrath JM, Mulder L, et al. Serum soluble interleukin-2 receptor measure-ment in patients with sarcoidosis: a clinical evaluation. *Chest.* 2003;124:186-95.

35. Judson MA. The diagnosis of sarcoidosis. *Clin Chest Med.* 2008;29:415-27, viii.

36. Carbone J, Perez-Rojas J, Sarmiento E. Infectious pulmonary complications in patients treated with anti-TNF-alfa monoclonal antibodies and soluble TNF receptor. *Curr Infect Dis Rep.* 2009;11:229-36.

37. Milman N, Burton CM, Iversen M, et al. Pulmonary hypertension in end-stage pulmonary sarcoidosis: therapeutic effect of sildenafil? *J Heart Lung Transplant.* 2008;27:329-34.

38. Handa T, Nagai S, Miki S, et al. Incidence of pulmonary hypertension and its clinical relevance in patients with sarcoidosis. *Chest.* 2006;129:1246-52.

39. Rizzato G, Pezzano A, Sala G, et al. Right heart impairment in sarcoidosis: haemodynamic and echocardiographic study. *Eur J Respir Dis.* 1983;64:121-8.

40. Diaz-Guzman E, Farver C, Parambil J, et al. Pulmonary hypertension caused by sarcoidosis. *Clin Chest Med.* 2008;29:549-63, x.

41. Baughman RP, Engel PJ, Meyer CA, et al. Pulmonary hypertension in sarcoidosis. *Sarcoidosis Vasc Diffuse Lung Dis.* 2006;23:108-16.

42. Newman LS, Rose CS, Bresnitz EA, et al. A case control etiologic study of sarcoidosis: environmental and occupational risk factors. *Am J Respir Crit Care Med.* 2004;170: 1324-30.

43. Winterbauer RH, Kirtland SH, Corley DE. Treatment with corticosteroids. *Clin Chest Med.* 1997;18:843-51.

44. De Remee RA. The present status of treatment of pulmonary sarcoidosis: a house divided. *Chest.* 1977;71:388-93.

45. Schutt AC, Bullington WM, Judson MA. Pharmacotherapy for pulmonary sarcoidosis: a delphi consensus study. *Respir Med.* 2010;104:717-23. Epub 2010 Jan 20.

46. Baughman RP, Winget DB, Lower EE. Methotrexate is steroid sparing in acute sarcoidosis: results of a double blind, randomized trial. *Sarcoidosis Vasc Diffuse Lung Dis.* 2000; 17:60-6.

47. Lower EE, Baughman RP. The use of low dose methotrexate in refractory sarcoidosis. *Am J Med Sci.* 1990;299:153-7.

48. Baughman RP, Lower EE. A clinical approach to the use of methotrexate for sarcoidosis. *Thorax.* 1999;54:742-6.

49. Baltzan M, Mehta S, Kirkham TH, et al. Randomized trial of prolonged chloroquine therapy in advanced pulmonary sarcoidosis. *Am J Respir Crit Care Med.* 1999;160:192-7.

50. Bartel PR, Roux P, Robinson E, et al. Visual function and long-term chloroquine treatment. *S Afr Med J.* 1994;84:32-4.

51. Muller-Quernheim J, Kienast K, Held M, et al. Treatment of chronic sarcoidosis with an azathioprine/prednisolone regimen. *Eur Respir J.* 1999;14:1117-22.

52. Lewis SJ, Ainslie GM, Bateman ED. Efficacy of azathioprine as second-line treatment in pulmonary sarcoidosis. *Sarcoidosis Vasc Diffuse Lung Dis.* 1999;16:87-92.

53. Zabel P, Entzian P, Dalhoff K, et al. Pentoxifylline in treatment of sarcoidosis. *Am J Respir Crit Care Med.* 1997;155:1665-9.

54. Judson MA, Silvestri J, Hartung C, et al. The effect of thalidomide on corticosteroid-dependent pulmonary sarcoidosis. *Sarcoidosis Vasc Diffuse Lung Dis.* 2006;23:51-7.

55. Rossman MD, Newman LS, Baughman RP, et al. A double-blinded, randomized, placebo-controlled trial of infliximab in subjects with active pulmonary sarcoidosis. *Sarcoidosis Vasc Diffuse Lung Dis.* 2006;23:201-8.

56. Baughman RP, Drent M, Kavuru M, et al. Infliximab therapy in patients with chronic sarcoidosis and pulmonary involvement. *Am J Respir Crit Care Med.* 2006;174:795-802.

57. Baughman RP, Judson MA, Teirstein A, et al. Presenting characteristics as predictors of duration of treatment in sarcoidosis. *QJM.* 2006;99:307-15. Epub 2006 Apr 4.

Acute Exacerbations of Hypersensitivity Pneumonitis

Lawrence Mohr

INTRODUCTION

Hypersensitivity pneumonitis (HP), also known as extrinsic allergic alveolitis, is a granulomatous, inflammatory disease of the lungs caused by the inhalation of organic dust particles. It is a multifaceted immunological disease that is triggered by immune complex-mediated (type III) hypersensitivity reactions and T cell mediated (type IV) hypersensitivity reactions that occur sequentially after inhalation of an inciting antigen. The pathogenesis of HP involves the inflammatory infiltration of lung tissue by CD8+ and CD4+ T-lymphocytes, the production of inflammatory cytokines, tumor necrosis factor-alfa (TNF-alfa), interferon-gamma (IFN-gamma), and specific precipitating antibodies against the inhaled antigen that triggers the immunological reactions.[1-6] It has been demonstrated that IFN-gamma is essential for the development of the disease.[4] HP is not associated with an increased number of eosinophils or the production of IgE. Therefore, it is not an allergic or atopic disorder, as the term allergic alveolitis might imply. Furthermore, the disease primarily involves the interstitium of the lung and is classified as an interstitial lung disease, although alveoli and the airways are often involved as well.[1]

Ramazini first recognized HP as a distinct clinical disorder in 1713, when he reported typical characteristics of the disease among wheat reapers.[7] Since that time, the disease has been associated with a wide variety of inhaled organic antigens. It has also been reported under a variety of descriptive names such as farmer's lung, silo filler's disease, bird fancier's lung, pigeon breeder's disease, bagassosis, and soybean lung. It is now understood that HP is a single disease entity that can be caused by different inhaled organic antigens. Affected individuals are genetically susceptible to the immunological effects caused by the inhalation of a specific inciting antigen. The disease is triggered upon inhalation of a specific inciting antigen by susceptible individuals[1,8] It has been reported that there is an increased frequency of HLA-DRB1*1305 and HLA-DQB1*0501 alleles among individuals with bird-related HP.[9,10] It has also been reported that individuals with HP have an increased frequency of the TNF-2-308 polymorphism of the TNF-alfa promoter gene, which is associated with a high level of TNF-alfa production.[1,10,11] Although these reports provide some insight into factors associated with genetic susceptibility to HP, additional studies are required to fully understand why some individuals are susceptible to developing HP following the inhalation of certain organic antigens while other individuals are not.

HP has acute, subacute, and chronic forms, all of which have been associated with acute exacerbations upon re-exposure to the inciting antigen. The lung inflammation which occurs in acute and subacute HP is primarily mediated by the Th1 cytokine network.[6,12] Both the Th1 and the Th2 cytokine networks contribute to the lung inflammation seen in chronic HP.[6,13]

EPIDEMIOLOGY

More than 300 different organic antigens have been associated with the development of HP. These antigens consist of plant products, animal products, aerosolized micro-organisms, and organic chemicals. Common inciting antigens are summarized in table 7-1.

The prevalence of HP in any given population is related to the specific organic antigens to which the population is exposed, antigen concentration, frequency and duration of antigen exposures, solubility of inhaled antigens, size of the particles containing the offending antigens, and the use of respiratory protection in the workplace.[1] It has been estimated that the prevalence of HP is between 5% and 15% of the overall population exposed to known inciting antigens.[14] Symptoms compatible

Table 7-1	Common Etiologic Antigens of Hypersensitivity Pneumonitis	
Antigen	*Source*	*Exposure risk*
Thermophilic actinomycetes	Moldy hay and compost	Farmers
Bacillus subtilis proteins	Contaminated wood dust	Woodworkers
Avian proteins	Bird droppings and feathers	Bird fanciers/pigeon breeders
Rodent proteins	Rodent dander	Animal handlers/lab workers
Amoeba (*Naegleria gruberi*)	Contaminated HVAC systems	Office workers
Penicillium sp.	Cheese mold	Cheese workers
Aspergillus sp.	Contaminated barley	Malt workers and brewers
Mycobacterium avium	Hot tubs	Hot tub users
Wheat weevil protein	Infected wheat	Wheat workers/silo fillers
Soybean hull antigens	Soybeans in animal feed	Farmers/animal feed handlers
Anhydrides	Plastic components	Plastic workers
Isocyanates	Paint hardeners	Painters

HVAC, heating, ventilation, and air conditioning.

with HP are seen in 5–10% of farmers and up to 15% of pigeon breeders.[15,16] It has also been reported that up to 70% of individuals exposed to microbe-contaminated air conditioning systems develop HP.[17] These data underscore the importance of individual genetic susceptibility in the development of HP, since only a fraction of individuals exposed to inhaled organic antigens actually develop the disease. Of interest is the fact that 95% of acute and subacute hypersensitivity pneumonitis cases occur in nonsmokers.[18] The lower incidence of acute and subacute HP among smokers may be related to a decrease in the production of specific precipitating antibodies to inhaled organic antigens due to the suppression of respiratory tract immunological responses by tobacco smoke.[1] Although smoking appears to protect against the development of acute and subacute HP, it has been demonstrated that smoking may contribute to the development and progression of chronic HP.[6,19,20]

The different clinical presentations of acute, subacute, and chronic HP most likely reflect differences in genetically controlled immunological responses in different individuals, as well as the frequency and extent of exposure to the inciting organic antigen. The clinical characteristics of each of the three types of HP, as well as the nature of the exacerbations that are associated with each type, are discussed in the following sections.

ACUTE HYPERSENSITIVITY PNEUMONITIS

Clinical Characteristics

The acute form of HP is the most common clinical presentation. It typically starts with influenza-like symptoms 4–8 hours after exposure to the inciting antigen. Specific symptoms include nonproductive cough, dyspnea, fever, chills, myalgias, and malaise. These symptoms typically reach peak intensity between 12 and 24 hours after exposure to the inciting antigen and resolve without specific treatment within 48 hours after cessation of exposure. On physical examination, the patient is ill appearing with tachypnea, tachycardia, and bibasilar inspiratory rales. Hypoxemia typically occurs and may range from mild to severe. The alveolar-arterial oxygen pressure gradient ($P[A-a]O_2$) is usually elevated. Cyanosis may occur in severely ill individuals with significant hypoxemia.

Although lung biopsy is usually not necessary to make the diagnosis of acute HP, the histopathology of this disorder has been well characterized. Typically, there is an inflammatory interstitial infiltrate consisting of lymphocytes, plasma cells, mast cells, and macrophages. CD4+ T-lymphocytes predominate initially, but CD8+ T-lymphocytes become the predominant inflammatory cell type during the first 24 hours. Neutrophils are usually found in the lumen of the airways during the first 48 hours following acute exposure to the inciting antigen.[1] Scattered, poorly formed, noncaseating granulomas, and multinucleated giant cells are frequently seen. The granulomas tend to be centilobular and adjacent to bronchioles.[1,21] Bronchiolitis and bronchiolitis obliterans with organizing pneumonia may be present in some cases.[1,22-25]

Diagnosis

Acute HP should be suspected in any patient who has an influenza-like illness with reticulonodular infiltrates or ground-glass opacities on a chest radiograph. The differential diagnosis includes atypical pneumonia, viral pneumonia, pulmonary edema, bronchoalveolar cell carcinoma, and organic toxic dust syndrome. The diagnosis of acute HP requires the presence of characteristic clinical features, a careful environmental and occupational history that establishes the association of symptoms with exposure to a known inciting antigen, the presence of specific precipitating antibodies to a known inciting antigen, and typical radiographic characteristics.

A high index of suspicion and a comprehensive, careful environmental and occupational history are the keys for making a correct diagnosis of acute HP. It is important that the history provides detailed information about the patient's work environment, home environment, pets, hobbies, travel, and similar illnesses among co-workers and family members.[1] When acute HP is suspected, every effort should be made to obtain historical information that correlates the onset of the symptoms with exposure to a known inciting antigen. It has been shown that the strongest single diagnostic predictor of HP is identification of exposure to a known inciting antibody.[26]

Serum precipitating antibodies to the inciting organic antigen, which are usually IgG but may be IgM or IgA, are almost always present during episodes of acute HP. The presence of precipitating antibodies is usually determined by Ouchterlony radial diffusion analysis. This technique involves exposing the patient's serum to one or more "panels" of specific organic antigens that are commonly related to the development of HP. The "panel" or "panels" of precipitating antibodies that are ordered by the physician should be guided by information obtained from the environmental and occupational history. This method of testing for precipitating antibodies is quite sensitive, and the absence of precipitating antibodies makes the diagnosis of acute HP unlikely. Unfortunately, such testing is not very specific, since precipitating antibodies to organic antigens are frequently found in exposed individuals who do not become ill.[27] Therefore, the presence of precipitating antibodies must be correlated with clinical symptoms and signs, the environmental and occupational history and with radiographic findings in order to establish the diagnosis of HP. Furthermore, the concentration of precipitating antibodies tends to decrease with disease progression and is also depressed by cigarette smoke. Consequently, there is no quantitative correlation between the concentration of precipitating antibodies and the severity of acute HP.[28-31]

Chest radiographs during episodes of acute HP typically show bilateral reti-culonodular infiltrates that may be either patchy or diffuse. These infiltrates tend to occur in the lower lung fields with sparing of the apices. On high resolution computed tomography (CT) scans of the chest, the infiltrates have a ground-glass appearance caused by the presence of multiple, clearly discernable micronodules.[32] A high resolution CT scan of a patient with acute hypersensitivity pneumonitis is shown in figure 7-1. The radiographic abnormalities of acute HP typically begin to resolve within five days after cessation of exposure, with radiographic clearing occurring between two and six weeks after the resolution of clinical symptoms. Both the chest radiograph and high resolution CT scans may be entirely normal between attacks.[33]

Pulmonary function tests during episodes of acute HP typically show restrictive ventilatory impairment, increased elastic recoil, decreased diffusion capacity, hypocapnia and hypoxemia that typically becomes more severe with exercise. The hypoxemia is usually characterized by an elevated $P[A-a]O_2$ gradient. Concurrent, and mild, obstructive ventilatory impairment occasionally occurs in some patients. The obstructive impairment may or may not have a reversible component following bronchodilator therapy. The presence of significant, reversible airway obstruction should suggest the possibility of occupational asthma, which occurs concurrently in 5–10% of patients with HP. The abnormal pulmonary function tests and arterial oxygen tension (PaO_2) typically return to normal between episodes of acute HP. Laboratory findings during episodes of acute HP typically include a neutrophilic leukocytosis, lymphopenia, and a normal IgE level in peripheral blood. Rheumatoid

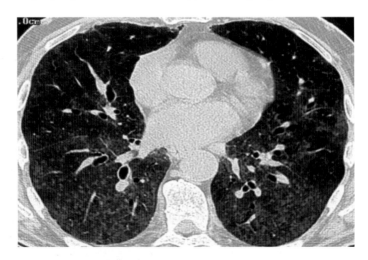

Figure 7-1 HRCT of acute hypersensitivity pneumonitis showing scattered ground-glass opacities consisting of multiple micronodules.

factor is positive in 50% of patients and nonspecific markers of inflammation, such as erythrocyte sedimentation rate and C-reactive protein, are frequently elevated. These laboratory abnormalities are nonspecific and typically return to normal between episodes of acute HP.

The presence of serum precipitating antibodies is usually sufficient to confirm the diagnosis of acute HP in a patient with a typical clinical course, history, and radiographic findings. In some cases, it can be useful to visit the suspected site of antigen exposure and have an industrial hygienist obtain, air, water, or soil samples for culture and chemical analysis in order to isolate a microbial organism or offending chemical. This approach is especially useful if multiple cases are reported from a single work site or residence.

Bronchoalveolar lavage (BAL) is not particularly useful for making the diagnosis of acute HP. For the first 24–48 hours after antigen exposure, an acute neutrophilic increase in cell count is seen in the lavage fluid. Approximately 48 hours after antigen exposure, lymphocytes begin to predominate.[8,34,35] The percentage of lymphocytes in the total cell count at this point in time tends to correlate with the degree of lung inflammation.[36,37] Furthermore, in acute HP the lymphocytes are predominately of the CD4+ subtype initially, but CD8+ lymphocytes eventually predominate as the acute disease progresses.[38,39] Between 24 and 48 hours after antigen exposure, plasma cells are typically seen in the lavage fluid, as well. In general, lavage fluid characteristics are quite variable in acute HP. The type of inciting antigen, the inhaled dose of the inciting antigen, the time after antigen exposure, and the presence of other nonspecific irritants all affect the characteristics of the lavage fluid at any given point in time. This high degree of variability makes it problematic to ascertain any specific diagnostic information from lavage fluid obtained during an episode of acute HP.

As previously mentioned, lung biopsy is usually not necessary to make the diagnosis of acute HP. It should be considered only if the clinical, historical, laboratory, and radiographic findings are insufficient to make a definitive diagnosis.[1]

Exacerbations

Episodes of acute HP typically recur whenever a susceptible individual inhales the inciting antigen. Between acute episodes, affected individuals are usually asymptomatic and feel entirely well. However, the severity of recurrent acute episodes tends to be greater than the severity of previous acute episodes. Thus, some individuals may experience relatively mild episodes at first, but recurrent episodes typically become progressively more severe over time. Patients who have experienced numerous recurrent episodes of acute HP may become severely ill with profound hypoxemia during subsequent recurrent episodes.

Treatment

Avoidance of exposure to the inciting antigen is the most important factor in the management of all forms of HP.[1,8,9,40] Patients with acute HP should be removed from the offending environment until symptoms have totally resolved. In most cases the illness is self-limited, with complete resolution of symptoms within 48 hours if re-exposure to the inciting antigen is avoided. Oral prednisone (40–60 mg per day) for 1–2 weeks, tapered over a period of 4–6 weeks, produces dramatic clinical and radiographic improvement in severe cases.[1,8,41,42] Oxygen should be administered if significant hypoxemia is present. Patients should be fitted for personal respiratory protection devices prior to returning to the offending environment if any possibility of antigen exposure still exists.[1,8,9,43] Environmental control measures, such as replacing filters on heating and air conditioning systems, changing humidifier water frequently, and improving air ventilation can help to prevent antigen exposure. In some cases, however, complete removal from the workplace or home may be necessary to entirely avoid exposure to an inciting antigen.[1,8]

SUBACUTE HYPERSENSITIVITY PNEUMONITIS

Clinical Characteristics

Repeated exposure to low doses of the inciting organic antigen can produce a subacute form of HP. Subacute HP is characterized by symptoms similar to those experienced by patients with chronic bronchitis. These include intermittent episodes of mild dyspnea, either at rest or on exertion, and occasional cough upon exposure to the inciting antigen. Low grade fever may occasionally occur. Symptoms typically resolve without treatment within 24 hours after cessation of exposure, but tend to recur shortly after re-exposure to a low dose of the inciting antigen. Mild hypoxemia with an elevated $P[A\text{-}a]O_2$ gradient may be present during symptomatic subacute episodes, but significant hypoxemia usually does not occur.[1]

Individuals with subacute HP typically feel entirely well during periods when they are not exposed to the inciting antigen. However, the symptoms experienced during each episode tend to be progressively more severe with repeated low-dose antigen exposures. Thus, the subacute form of HP is typically characterized by frequent episodes of nonspecific respiratory symptoms that become progressively more severe with repeated low-dose exposures to the inciting antigen over a period of many years. Chronic fatigue and weight loss may occur in patients with frequent subacute episodes.[40]

The histopathological characteristics of subacute HP have been well defined. The most characteristic feature is the presence of scattered, well-formed, epithelioid granulomas, similar to those seen in sarcoidosis. However, the granulomas seen in subacute HP are centrilobular, whereas the granulomas seen in sarcoidosis are peribronchovascular; this is an important pathological distinction between the two diseases. A minimal mononuclear cell infiltrate, with cell types similar to those seen in acute HP, is typically seen. The extent of the interstitial infiltrate is variable and probably depends upon the inhaled dose of the inciting antigen, as well as the time interval between repeated exposures. Most importantly, the interstitial infiltrate occurs both adjacent to and distant from the granulomas. This can also be helpful in differentiating subacute HP from sarcoidosis, in which the interstitial infiltrates typically occur adjacent to the granulomas.[1]

Diagnosis

Given the mild and nonspecific respiratory symptoms that are typically associated with subacute HP, this form of the disease can be problematic to diagnose. Affected individuals may not seek medical attention until their episodic symptoms become severe enough to interfere with daily activities. This may preclude the possibility of making a timely diagnosis early in the course of the disease. As with acute HP, the keys to making a correct diagnosis of subacute HP are a high index of suspicion and a careful, systematic environmental, and occupational history.

Serum precipitating antibodies to the specific inciting antigen are almost always present in individuals with subacute HP. The presence of specific serum precipitating antibodies can be very helpful in making the diagnosis of subacute HP when correlated with the clinical, historical, and radiographic findings.

The chest radiograph may be normal during episodes of subacute HP but fine micronodules may be evident after years of recurrent subacute episodes. These micronodules are readily visible on high resolution CT scans of the chest. The micronodules are caused by persistent granulomas that form as a result of chronic low-grade inflammation associated with frequent, low-dose antigen exposures. They do not resolve between subacute episodes. A high resolution CT scan of a patient with subacute HP is shown in figure 7-2.

Pulmonary function tests typically show minimal restrictive ventilatory impairment, with or without impairment of diffusion capacity, and with or without mild hypoxemia, during symptomatic subacute episodes. As in the acute form of HP, pulmonary function tests and PaO_2 may be normal between subacute episodes. Laboratory tests are typically normal, although variable degrees of lymphopenia may occur in some patients.

BAL may be helpful in confirming the diagnosis of subacute HP that cannot be made with certainty from available clinical, historical, laboratory, and radiographic information. Bronchoalveolar lavage fluid typically shows a 3–5-fold increase in cell count with an elevated percentage of lymphocytes, typically in the range of 30–70%.[44] Most importantly, most lymphocytes are T-lymphocytes that express the CD8+ antigen. As a result, the CD4+/CD8+ T-lymphocyte ratio in the lavage

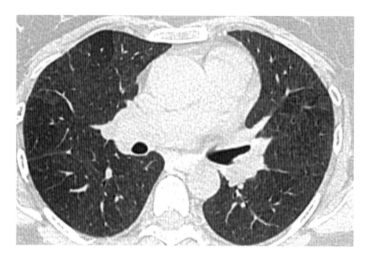

Figure 7-2 HRCT of subacute hypersensitivity pneumonitis showing multiple micronodules and scattered areas of early fibrosis.

fluid is typically less than one.[42,45] This can be particularly helpful in distinguishing subacute HP from sarcoidosis, in which the CD4+/CD8+ ratio in lavage fluid is typically greater than 1 and usually greater than 3.5. A recent report demonstrates that approximately 10% of the lymphocytes in the lavage fluid of individuals with subacute HP expressed natural killer T-cell (NKT cell) markers, whereas approximately 3% of lymphocytes in the lavage fluid of individuals with sarcoidosis expressed NKT cell markers.[45] This was a statistically significant difference and suggests that assessment of NKT markers on lavage fluid lymphocytes may also be a helpful in differentiating subacute HP from sarcoidosis. Neutrophils may be seen in the lavage fluid of individuals with subacute HP within the first 48 hours following an acute exposure. Therefore, ascertaining the time of antigen exposure is helpful in interpreting the lavage fluid analysis.[46] Elevated concentrations of IgG, IgM, and IgA antibodies may also be found in the lavage fluid of individuals with subacute HP.[47-48]

Lung biopsy is usually not necessary to make the diagnosis of subacute HP and should only be considered if the diagnosis cannot be made with certainty by other means. The presence of well-formed centrilobular epitheloid granulomas with mononuclear cell interstitial infiltrates that are both adjacent to and distant from the granulomas can be helpful in distinguishing subacute HP from sarcoidosis; if a definitive diagnosis cannot be made by an environmental and occupational history, the presence of serum precipitating antibodies, radiographic characteristics, and bronchoalveolar lavage.

Exacerbations

Patients with subacute HP typically feel well during periods when they are not exposed to the inciting organic antigen. However, the symptoms experienced during each episode tend to become progressively more severe with repeated low-dose exposures. Similarly, pulmonary function tests typically show a progressive restrictive ventilatory impairment and a decline in diffusion capacity over time with recurrent subacute episodes. Some patients may have intermittent episodes of fulminant acute HP interspersed with recurrent episodes of subacute symptoms.[1] On high resolution CT scans of the chest, patients with acute exacerbations of subacute HP typically have new ground-glass opacities in the mid to lower lung fields that are superimposed on the fine micronodules of subacute HP. As occurs in acute HP, the ground-glass opacities typically resolve with cessation of antigen exposure.

Individuals who have recurrent episodes of symptomatic, subacute HP over a period of many years are at high risk of developing chronic HP.[1] The presence of micronodules on chest radiograph or high resolution CT scan, progressive restrictive ventilatory impairment, progressive decline in diffusion capacity, or progressive decline in SaO_2 during exercise should suggest the development of chronic HP in patients with a history of recurrent subacute episodes.[1,49]

Treatment

As with other forms of HP, the mainstay of treatment for subacute HP is avoidance of exposure to the inciting antigen. Cessation of exposure to the inciting antigen usually results in complete resolution of subacute HP symptoms within 24 hours. Complete avoidance of recurrent or continuous low-dose antigen exposure is helpful in preventing the progression of subacute HP to chronic HP and is an important consideration in the management of patients with subacute HP.[1,8,9]

Oral corticosteroids should be considered for the treatment of subacute HP episodes that do not resolve within 24 hours after cessation of antigen exposure or for intermittent exacerbations of acute HP that occur in patients with a history of subacute HP. Prednisone (40–60 mg per day) for 1–2 weeks, tapered over a period of 4–6 weeks, is a reasonable regimen in such cases.[1,8,41,42] Oxygen should be administered as necessary to maintain the SaO_2 greater than 90%.

CHRONIC HYPERSENSITIVITY PNEUMONITIS

Clinical Characteristics

Approximately 5% of patients with HP develop the chronic form of the disease.[1,7] Chronic HP is a debilitating disease characterized by progressive, irreversible pulmonary fibrosis. The pulmonary fibrosis develops insidiously over a period of months to years in susceptible individuals who have continuous or frequent exposure to the inciting antigen. Recurrent episodes of subacute HP often herald the development of chronic disease.

The symptoms of chronic HP resemble those of advanced chronic bronchitis, including persistent progressive cough, mucus production, dyspnea on exertion, weight loss, anorexia, and malaise. Fever is rare. Tachypnea and bibasilar crackles are usually present on physical examination. Signs of cor pulmonale may be present in severe cases.[1] The five year mortality rate is in the range of 10–30%.[50-53] Therefore, chronic hypersensitivity can be a life-threatening disease, especially if it is associated with the development of cor pulmonale.

The histopathological features of chronic HP have overlapping patterns of usual interstitial pneumonia (UIP) and nonspecific interstitial pneumonitis (NSIP). One of these two histopathological patterns tends to dominate in most individuals with chronic HP. Both patterns are characterized by peribronchiolar, lymphocyte-predominant, interstitial infiltrates. Centrilobular fibrosis is commonly found and granulomas may or may not be present.[6,54-59] In general, as chronic HP increases in severity, pulmonary fibrosis predominates and granulomas tend to disappear. Areas of organizing pneumonia, with or without coexisting bronchiolitis, may be seen in both major histopathological patterns of chronic HP.

Diagnosis

Establishing the diagnosis of chronic HP requires that other fibrotic, interstitial lung diseases are excluded from the differential diagnosis, particularly UIP and NSIP. Because chronic HP can closely resemble these other interstitial lung diseases, making the correct diagnosis can be challenging, even for the most experienced clinicians.

As with the acute and subacute forms of HP, a high index of suspicion and a careful environmental and occupational history are important for guiding the medical evaluation and making the correct diagnosis. It is particularly important to obtain a history of previous episodes that are consistent with acute or subacute HP, the number of months or years during which the episodes occurred, the frequency of such episodes, and exposure to any potential antigen sources that were associated with the onset of previous episodes.

The demonstration of serum precipitating antibodies to antigens associated with previous acute and subacute episodes may be helpful in making the diagnosis of chronic HP. However, the presence of serum precipitating antibodies does exclude other interstitial lung diseases, since precipitating antibodies only reflect previous exposure to a specific antigen and do not, by themselves, establish a definitive diagnosis of HP.[27,28,40,60-62] Furthermore, as chronic HP progresses, titers of precipitating antibodies tend to decrease and may eventually become undetectable. It is also possible that some individuals with chronic HP no longer have contact with the inciting antigen, since their chronic illness precludes them from working or engaging in hobbies in those environments in which exposure to the inciting antigen took place. Removal from antigen exposure could also result in a decrease, or absence, of serum precipitating antibodies. Thus, the absence of serum precipitating antibodies does not exclude the possibility of chronic HP.[1,28-31] If present, serum precipitating antibodies must be correlated with the clinical, historical, pathological, and radiographic findings to have intrinsic diagnostic value.

Chronic HP is characterized by progressive, irreversible, and fibrotic lung damage. Radiographically, this is manifested by small lung volumes, scattered areas of honeycombing and diffuse reticulonodular infiltrates in the mid to lower lung fields. High resolution CT scans show findings similar to idiopathic pulmonary fibrosis, with foci of interstitial fibrosis, patchy ground-glass opacities, traction bronchiectasis and multiple centrilobular nodules measuring 2–4 mm in diameter.[1,63] While these radiographic findings tend to predominate in the mid to lower lung fields, the lung bases are usually spared in chronic HP.[64-66] Well-demarcated areas of increased radiolucency can often be seen among ground-glass opacities and are thought to represent hyperinflated pulmonary lobules caused by partially obstructed bronchioles. It has been reported that the mortality of patients with chronic HP increases with the extent of radiographic fibrosis.[52,67] Unlike the acute form of HP, radiographic findings do not resolve completely with cessation of exposure to the inciting antigen. A high resolution computed tomography scan of a patient with chronic HP is shown in figure 7-3.

Individuals with chronic HP typically have pulmonary function tests that show progressive restrictive ventilatory impairment, with a reduction in lung volumes,

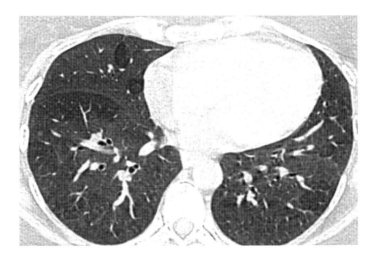

Figure 7-3 HRCT of chronic hypersensitivity pneumonitis showing subpleural interstitial fibrosis with areas of honeycombing and areas of traction bronchiectasis.

increased elastic recoil and decreased diffusion capacity. Mild obstructive ventilatory impairment may occur, but this is unusual in chronic HP and is typically irreversible when present. It has been reported that the patients with increased FEV_1/FVC ratios have a higher mortality. In patients with chronic HP, a high FEV1/FVC ratio can be caused by increased elastic recoil of the lung and/or a decrease in airway resistance, both of which are a consequence of lung tissue fibrosis. Patients with lower oxygen saturations during exercise also have a higher mortality rate.[52,67,68] The pulmonary function abnormalities of chronic HP do not return to normal with cessation of exposure to the inciting antigen.

BAL can be useful in distinguishing chronic HP from other chronic interstitial lung diseases, particularly idiopathic pulmonary fibrosis (IPF) and stage IV sarcoidosis. BAL is less useful in distinguishing chronic HP from NSIP, since there is considerable overlap in cell counts and cell types in both diseases.[1,69,70] As with subacute HP, the lavage fluid will usually show an increased cell count, with an elevated percentage of lymphocytes in the range of 30–70%. However, recent reports demonstrate that the ratio of CD4+/CD8+ T-lymphocytes has considerable variability in chronic HP, and may not be less than 1, as it is in the subacute form of the disease.[71-74] This variability is related to the fact that activity of the Th1 cytokine network declines and activity of the Th2 cytokine network increases as the fibrosis of chronic HP progresses. Although the specific reasons for this change in cytokine network activity are currently unknown, it is clear that the shift from Th1 to Th2 cytokine activity promotes the fibrotic process by the induction of fibroblast proliferation and collagen production. The shift from Th1 to Th2 cytokine activity also favors the production and proliferation of CD4+ T-lymphocytes rather than CD8+ T-lymphocytes.[71,75,76] As a result, the CD4+/CD8+ T-lymphocyte ratio may become greater than one as the fibrosis of chronic HP progresses.[38,71] It is clear, however, that an elevated total lymphocyte count in the lavage fluid of patient with a chronic interstitial lung disease of uncertain etiology should prompt the clinician to carefully consider the diagnosis of chronic HP, that a CD4+/CD8+ lymphocyte ratio of less than one favors the diagnosis of chronic HP, and that a normal total lymphocyte count in the lavage fluid essentially excludes the diagnosis of chronic HP.[40,77-79] As in subacute HP, assessment of natural killer T-cell markers (NKT markers) on lavage fluid lymphocytes may prove to be helpful in differentiating chronic HP from other chronic interstitial lung diseases, particularly sarcoidosis.[45]

Because of the potential difficulty in distinguishing chronic HP from other chronic interstitial lung diseases, a lung biopsy is often necessary to make the diagnosis with certainty. Transbronchial biopsies are adequate in most cases.[1] Although some reports suggest that surgical lung biopsies may have a greater diagnostic yield, they are associated with increased morbidity and there is no evidence that they significantly alter clinical management.[40] Therefore, it is generally recommended that surgical biopsies be reserved for cases of suspected chronic HP that are particularly problematic, or for cases in which the clinical course or response to therapy is distinctly unusual.[40,80]

As previously mentioned, the histopathological characteristics of chronic HP have overlapping characteristics of UIP and NSIP, with one of these patterns tending to dominate in any given case. These are referred to as UIP-like and NSIP-like patterns, respectively. Areas of organizing pneumonia may be seen in both histopathological patterns, but it is not common for organizing pneumonia to be the predominant histopathological finding.

The UIP-like histopathological pattern is characterized by patchy perilobular fibrosis in the subpleural area and along the intralobular septa. Honeycomb changes are commonly seen in subpleural regions and areas of centrilobular fibrosis may be noted. Areas of constrictive bronchiolitis are commonly seen. Variable degrees of lymphocytic and plasma cell interstitial infiltration are present, but epitheloid granulomas are rare.[6] Consistent with commonly observed radiographic findings, most pathological changes are found in the mid to lower lung zones, although the lung bases are characteristically spared. The UIP-like histopathological pattern is most often seen in cases of chronic HP that have a slow, insidious onset, usually with recurrent episodes of subacute HP, over a period of many years.[6,81]

The NSIP-like histopathological pattern is characterized by mononuclear cell infiltration of the alveolar walls, bronchiolar walls, and intralobular septa, primarily with lymphocytes and plasma cells. Patchy areas of alveolar wall fibrosis and fibrosis of the intralobular septa are typically seen.[6] As with bronchoalveolar lavage findings, the histopathological characteristics of NSIP-like chronic HP can be virtually identical to NSIP, *per se.*[1] In such cases, the environmental and occupational history, the characteristics of previous acute and subacute episodes, and the presence of serum precipitating antibodies can be helpful in making the correct diagnosis. Consistent with typical radiographic findings, the histopathological changes are primarily seen in the mid to lower lung zones, with sparing of the lung bases. NSIP-like chronic HP is most often seen in patients that have a history of recurrent episodes of acute HP.[81] Laboratory findings in individuals with chronic HP are similar to those found in acute and subacute disease, including neutrophilic leukocytosis, lymphopenia, and a normal IgE level in peripheral blood.

Exacerbations

As seen in other chronic interstitial lung diseases, individuals with chronic HP may experience acute exacerbations.[6,82-85] The primary symptoms of an acute exacerbation are the onset of rapidly increasing dyspnea and persistent nonproductive cough that develop over a period of several weeks to several months. The progressive increase in dyspnea is typically associated with a progressive decline in pulmonary function and oxygenation. Patients who experience acute exacerbations of chronic HP have a high mortality rate, despite aggressive treatment with high-dose corticosteroids and other anti-inflammatory drugs. Reported mortality rates are in the range of 75–95%.[82-84] The cause of acute exacerbations is not known but they do not appear to be directly associated with re-exposure to the offending antigen. An acute exacerbation of chronic HP can occur at any time in the course of the disease.[82,84,85]

Although it is not possible to predict with certainty which patients with chronic HP will experience acute exacerbations, it has been shown that acute exacerbations tend to occur in males, in patients with a history of smoking, and in those with a UIP-like histological pattern on lung biopsy. It has been reported that 11.5% of patients with UIP-like chronic HP develop acute exacerbations.[83] Acute exacerbations have been reported in patients with an NSIP-like histopathological pattern, but the incidence is much lower in comparison to the incidence of acute exacerbations in those with a UIP-like pattern. It has also been reported that patients who develop acute exacerbations of chronic HP have lower baseline total lung capacities (TLC) and lower diffusion capacities in comparison to patients who do not have acute exacerbations.[82,83]

On high resolution computed tomography of the chest, acute exacerbations of chronic HP are typically characterized by new bilateral ground-glass opacities overlying areas of chronic interstitial fibrosis. Areas of traction bronchiectasis, which are frequently seen in cases of chronic HP, may be seen among the ground-glass opacities. The extent and density of the ground-glass opacities correlate with the degree of increased dyspnea that is experienced by the patient. A high resolution computed tomography scan of a patient with an acute exacerbation of chronic HP is shown in figure 7-4.[84]

The primary pulmonary function abnormality in acute exacerbations of chronic HP is a progressive impairment in gas exchange. This is manifested by a progressive decline in PaO_2, increase in the $P[A-a]O_2$ gradient, decline in SaO_2 at rest and during exercise, and a decline in diffusion capacity. Most reported cases of acute exacerbations of chronic HP eventually developed hypoxemic respiratory failure that required mechanical ventilatory support and eventually resulted in death in spite of aggressive treatment.[82-84]

Lung biopsies of patients with acute exacerbations of chronic HP have been reported to show diffuse alveolar damage (DAD), with or without concomitant areas of organizing pneumonia, in conjunction with interstitial and peribronchiolar fibrosis. Giant cells and alveolar hyaline membranes may also be seen, but epitheloid granulomas are rare. As previously stated, most acute exacerbations occur in patients who have an underlying UIP-like histological pattern of chronic HP. In this group of patients, the clinical characteristics, radiographic findings, and pathological findings of acute exacerbation of chronic HP are similar to those found in patients with UIP itself.[82,83,85,86]

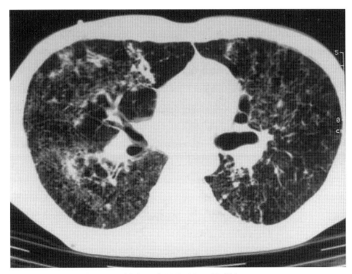

Image courtesy: Dr Anand Jaiswal, MD, New Delhi

Figure 7-4 HRCT of acute exacerbation of chronic hypersensitivity pneumonitis showing dense ground-glass opacities overlying interstitial fibrosis with areas of subpleural honeycombing. Traction bronchiectasis is also seen.

Treatment

The prognosis of chronic HP depends upon the extent of permanent lung damage at the time of diagnosis. The majority of patients with mild chronic disease show some improvement in both pulmonary function and radiographic abnormalities with complete avoidance of the inciting antigen. These patients may reach a functional plateau that requires no further therapy as long as they are not re-exposed to the antigen. In contrast, patients who develop advanced fibrosis tend to have continued progression of their disease, even with complete avoidance of re-exposure to the inciting antigen.[1,8] Such patients are likely to have a progressive deterioration of lung function leading to cor pulmonale, respiratory failure, and death.[8,29,87,88]

Although there are no controlled clinical trials regarding the treatment of patients with chronic HP, it is generally recommended that patients with severe or progressive disease be treated with a trial of oral corticosteroids. A reasonable regimen consists of prednisone (40–60 mg per day) for 4 weeks, slowly tapered to the lowest dose that is effective in ameliorating symptoms, which is usually in the range of 10–30 mg per day, over a period of 3 months. Therapy should then be continued at the lowest effective dose for an additional 2 months. After 6 months of therapy the patient should be evaluated with a clinical examination, pulmonary function tests, and radiographic studies. Therapy should be continued beyond 6 months only if an objective response can be documented.[1,89] Continuous oxygen therapy should be administered, as necessary, to maintain the SaO_2 greater than 90%.

It is generally recommended that acute exacerbations of chronic HP be treated with high-dose systemic corticosteroids initially. Intravenous methylprednisolone, 1000 mg per day for three days is generally recommended. This is followed by oral prednisone (0.5–1 mg/kg) that is gradually tapered to the lowest dose that ameliorates symptoms or to discontinuation over a period of 4–8 weeks. Cyclophosphamide and cyclosporine have both been used in addition to corticosteroids for the treatment of refractory exacerbations.[82,83] Although there are no controlled clinical trials to guide the therapy for acute exacerbations of chronic HP, aggressive therapy is highly recommended in view of the high mortality rate. Continuous oxygen therapy should be given as needed to maintain the SaO_2 greater than 90%. Some patients will require mechanical ventilation for the management of respiratory failure.[83,84] There is a single case report of a patient with a severe acute exacerbation who survived following bilateral lung transplantation.[84] Thus, it is reasonable to consider lung transplantation for suitable patients with severe acute exacerbations who develop refractory respiratory failure despite aggressive pharmacological therapy.

SUMMARY

HP is a multifaceted immunological disorder that is triggered after inhalation of an inciting organic antigen by a genetically susceptible individual. HP can present in acute, subacute, and chronic forms. Each of these three distinct forms of HP has characteristic clinical, radiographic, laboratory, and histopathological findings, although there can be an overlap of some characteristics in patients who are progressing from subacute to chronic disease as a result of repeated or continuous low-level exposure to the inciting antigen. The keys to making the correct diagnosis of HP, whether acute, subacute, or chronic, are a high index of suspicion and a careful environmental and occupational history.

Episodes of acute and subacute HP usually resolve soon after the patient ceases to have contact with the inciting antigen, although a course of oral corticosteroids may be needed in severe cases. Patients with chronic HP should also be removed from contact with the inciting antigen; however, patients with advanced fibrotic disease may experience progressive deterioration in pulmonary function even if they are no longer subjected to antigen exposure. It is recommended that all patients with severe or progressive chronic HP be treated with a six-month trial of oral corticosteroids. Corticosteroids should be continued beyond six months only if objective improvement in the clinical course, radiographic findings, or pulmonary function tests is documented.

Acute exacerbations may occur among individuals with each form of HP. Acute exacerbations in patients with acute and subacute HP typically occur after re-exposure to an inciting antigen and usually resolve soon after the patient is removed from antigen contact. Acute exacerbations of chronic HP do not appear to be associated with re-exposure to the inciting antigen, may be associated with severe hypoxemia, have a high mortality rate, should be treated aggressively with high-dose systemic corticosteroids, and may require mechanical ventilation for the management of respiratory failure. Lung transplantation should be considered for suitable patients who continue to deteriorate in spite of aggressive pharmacological therapy.

REFERENCES

1. Mohr LC. Hypersensitivity pneumonitis. *Curr Opin Pulm Med.* 2004;10:401-11.
2. Fink JN. Hypersensitivity pneumonitis. *Chest.* 1992;13:303-9.
3. Gudmundsson G, Monick MM, Hunninghake GW. IL-12 modulates expression of hypersensitivity pneumonitis. *J Immunol.* 1998;161:991-9.
4. Gudmundsson G, Hunninghake GW. Interferon-gamma is necessary for the expression of hypersensitivity pneumonitis. *J Clin Invest.* 1997;99:2386-90.
5. Ye Q, Nakimura S, Sarria R, et al. Interleukin 12, interleukin 18, and tumor necrosis factor release by alveolar macrophages: acute and chronic hypersensitivity pneumonitis. *Ann Allergy Asthma Immunol.* 2009;102:149-54.
6. Takemura T, Akashi T, Ohtani Y, et al. Pathology of hypersensitivity pneumonitis. *Curr Opin Pulm Med.* 2008;14:440-54.
7. Pozzi E. Extrinsic allergic alveolitis (hypersensitivity pneumonitis). In: Grassi C, Brambella C, Costabel U, Stockley RA, Naeije R, Rodriguez-Roisin R (Eds): *Pulmonary Diseases.* London: McGraw-Hill International (UK) Ltd;1999. pp 289-94.
8. Ismail T, McSharry C, Boyd G. Extrinsic allergic alveolitis. *Respirology.* 2006;11:262-8.
9. Selman M. Hypersensitivity pneumonitis: a multifaceted deceiving disorder. *Clin Chest Med.* 2004;25:521-47.
10. Camarena A, Juarez A, Mejia M, et al. Major histocompatibility complex and tumor necrosis factor- alfa polymorphisms in pigeon breeders disease. *Am J Respir Crit Care Med.* 201;163:1528-33.
11. Schaaf BM, Seitzer V, Pravica V, et al. Tumor necrosis factor-alfa-309 promoter gene polymorphism and increases tumor necrosis factor serum bioavailability in farmer's lung patients. *Am J Respir Crit Care Med.* 2001;163:379-82.
12. Ando M, Suga M, Kohrog H. A new look at hypersensitivity pneumonitis. *Curr Opin Pulm Med.* 1999;5:299-304.
13. Saibai T, Tanaka H, Sato N, et al. Mushroom plant workers experience a shift towards T helper type 2 dominant state: contribution of innate immunity to spore antigen. *Clin Exp Immunol.* 2004;135:119-24.
14. Lopez M, Salvage JE. Epidemiology of hypersensitivity pneumonitis/allergic alveolitis. *Monogram Allergy.* 1987;21:70-86.
15. Marx JJ, Guernsey J, Emanuel DA, et al. Cohort studies of immunologic lung disease among Wisconsin dairy farmers. *Am J Ind Med.* 1990;181:263-8.
16. Christensen LT, Schmidt CD, Robbins L. Pigeon breeders' disease: a prevalence study and review. *Clin Allergy.* 1975;5:417-30.
17. Hodgson MJ, Morey PR, Simon JS, et al. An outbreak of recurrent acute and chronic hypersensitivity pneumonitis in office workers. *Am J Epidemiol.* 1987;125:631-8.
18. Cormier Y, Gagnon L, Berube-Genest F, Fournier M. Extrinsic allergic alveolitis: the influence of cigarette smoking. *Am Rev Respir Dis.* 1988;137:1104-9.

19. Arima K, Ando M, Ito K, et al. Effect of cigarette smoking on prevalence of summer-type hypersensitivity pneumonitis caused by Tricosporon cutaneum. *Arch Environ Health.* 1992;47:274-8.

20. Ohtsuka Y, Munakata M, Tanimura K, et al. Smoking promotes insidious and chronic farmer's lung disease, deteriorates the clinical outcome. *Intern Med.* 1995;34:966-71.

21. Coleman A, Colby TV. Histologic diagnosis of extrinsic allergic alveolitis. *Am J Surg Path.* 1989;12:514-8.

22. Selman M, Vargas MH. Airway involvement in hypersensitivity pneumonitis. *Curr Opin Pulm Med.* 1998;4:9-15.

23. Reyes CN, Wenzel FJ, Lawton BR, et al. The pulmonary pathology of farmer's lung disease. *Chest.* 1982;81:142-6.

24. Wright JL. Inhalational lung injury causing bronchiolitis. *Clin Chest Med.* 1993;14:635-44.

25. Ryu JH, Myers JL, Swenson SJ. Bronchiolar disorders. *Am J Respir Crit Care Med.* 2003; 168:1277-92.

26. Lacasse Y, Selman M, Costabel V, et al. Clinical diagnosis of hypersensitivity pneumonitis. *Am J Respir Crit Care Med.* 2003;168:952-8.

27. Fink JN, Barboriak J, Sosman A, et al. Antibodies against pigeon serum proteins in pigeon breeders. *J Lab Clin Med.* 1968;71:20-4.

28. Baldwin CI, Todd A, Bourke A, et al. Pigeon fanciers' lung: effects of smoking on serum and salivary antibody responses to pigeon antigens. *Clin Exp Immunol.* 1998;113:166-72.

29. Barbee RA, Callies Q, Dickie HA, et al. The long-term prognosis in farmer's lung. *Am Rev Respir Dis.* 1968;97:223-31.

30. Gariepy L, Cormier Y, Laviolette M, et al. Predictive value of BAL cells and serum precipitins in asymptomatic dairy farmers. *Am Rev Respir Dis.* 1989;140:1386-9.

31. McSharry C, Anderson K, Bourke SJ, et al. Takes your breath away – the immunology of allergic alveolitis. *Clin Exp Immunol.* 2002;128:3-9.

32. Lynch DA, Newell JD, Logan PM, et al. Can CT distinguish hypersensitivity pneumonitis from idiopathic pulmonary fibrosis? *Am J Roentgenol.* 1995;165:807-11.

33. Hansell DM, Moskovic E. High-resolution computed tomography in extrinsic allergic alveolitis. *Clin Radiol.* 1991;43:8-12.

34. Costabel U, Bross KJ, Marten J, Mathis MD. T-lymphocytes in bronchoalveolar lavage fluid of hypersensitivity pneumonitis. Changes in profile of T-cell subsets during the course of disease. *Chest.* 1984;85:514-22.

35. Drent M, Van VelzenBlad H, Diamont M, et al. Bronchoalveolar lavage in extrinsic allergic alveolitis: effect of time elapses since antigen exposure. *Eur Respir J.* 1993;6:1276-81.

36. Trentin L, Marcer G, Chilosi M, et al. Longitudinal study of alveolitis in hypersensitivity patients: an immunological evaluation. *J Allergy Clin Immunol.* 1988;82:577-85.

37. Reynolds SP, Jones KP. Edwards JH, Davies BH. Inhalation challenge in pigeon breeders disease. BAL fluid changes after 6 hours. *Eur Respir J.* 1993;6:467-76.

38. Ohtani Y, Hisauchi K, Sumi Y, et al. Sequential changes in bronchoalveolar lavage cells and cytokines in a patient progressing from acute to chronic bird fanciers lung disease. *Intern Med.* 1999;38:896-9.

39. Reynolds SP, Jones KP, Edwards JH, Davies BH. Immunoregulatory proteins in bronchoalveolar lavage fluid. A comparative analysis of pigeon breeders' disease, sarcoidosis and idiopathic pulmonary fibrosis. *Sarcoidosis.* 1989;6:125-34.

40. Girard M, Lacasse Y, Cormier Y. Hypersensitivity pneumonitis. *Allergy.* 2009;64:322-34.

41. Karjalainen A, Martikainen R, Klaukka T. The risk of asthma among Finnish patients with farmer's lung. *Arch Occup Environ Health.* 2002;75:587-90.

42. Patel AM, Ryu JH, Reed CE. Hypersensitivity pneumonitis: current concepts and future questions. *J Allergy Clin Immunol.* 2001;108:661-70.

43. Anderson K, Walker A, Boyd G. The long-term effect of a positive pressure ventilator on the specific antibody response in pigeon breeders. *Clin Exp Allergy.* 1989;19:45-9.

44. Drent M, Mulder PGH, Wagwnaar SS, et al. Differences in BAL fluid variables in interstitial lung diseases evaluated by discriminant analysis. *Eur Respir J.* 1993;6:803-10.

45. Korosec P, Osolnik K, Kern I, et al. Expansion of pulmonary CD8+CD56+ natural killer T-cells in hypersensitivity pneumonitis. *Chest.* 2007;132:1291-7.

46. Fournier E, Tonnel AB, Gossett P, et al. Early neutrophil alveolitis after inhalation in hypersensitivity pneumonitis. *Chest.* 1985;88:563-6.

47. Calvanico NJ, Ambegaonkar SP, Schlueter DP, et al. Immunoglobulin levels in bronchoalveolar lavage fluid from pigeon breeders. *J Lab Clin Med.* 1980;96:129-40.

48. Reynolds SP, Edwards JH, Jones KP, et al. Immunoglobulin and antibody levels in bronchoalveolar lavage from symptomatic and asymptomatic pigeon breeders. *Clin Exp Immunol.* 1991;86:278-85.

49. Salvaggio JE. Extrinsic allergic alveolitis (hypersensitivity pneumonitis): past, present and future. *Clin Exp Allergy.* 1997;27:18-25.

50. Braun SR, DoPico GA, Tsiatis A, et al. Farmer's lung disease: long-term clinical and physiologic outcome. *Am Rev Respir Dis.* 1979;119:185-91.

51. Kokkarinen J, Tukiainen H, Tehro EO. Mortality due to farmer's lung in Finland. *Chest.* 1994;106:509-12.

52. Lima MS, Coletta EN, Ferreira BG, et al. Subacute and chronic hypersensitivity pneumonitis: Histopathological patterns and survival. *Respir Med.* 2009;103:508-15.

53. Perez-Padilla R, Salas J, Chapela R, et al. Mortality in Mexican patients with chronic pigeon breeder's lung compared with those with usual interstitial pneumonia. *Am Rev Respir Dis.* 1993;148:49-53.

54. Jacobs RL. Hypersensitivity pneumonia: UIP/IPF histopathologic presentation. *J Allergy Clin Immunol.* 2002;24:19-33.

55. Vourlekis JS, Schwarz MI, Cool CD, et al. Nonspecific interstitial pneumonitis as the sole histologic expression of hypersensitivity pneumonitis. *Am J Med.* 2002;112:490-3.

56. Hayakawa H, Shirai M, Sato A, et al. Clinicopathological features of hypersensitivity pneumonitis. *Respirology.* 2002;7:359-64.

57. Ohtani Y, Saiki S, Kitaichi M, et al. Chronic bird fancier's lung : histopathological and clinical correlation : an application of the 2002 ATS/ERS consensus classification of the idiopathic interstitial pneumonias. *Thorax.* 2005;60:665-71.

58. Churg A, Müller NL, Flint J, et al. Chronic hypersensitivity pneumonitis. *Am J Surg Path.* 2006;30:201-8.

59. Takemura T, Akashi T, Oritsu M, et al. Pathologic features of chronic hypersensitivity pneumonia – viewpoint of histogenesis from biopsy and autopsy lungs [abstract]. In: 4th International WASOG Conference; 2007. pp 26-7.

60. McSharry C, Anderson K, Bourke SJ, et al. Antibody measurement in extrinsic allergic alveolitis. *Eur J Respir Dis.* 1984;65:259-65.

61. Cormier Y, Belanger J, Beaudoin J, et al. Abnormal bronchoalveolar lavage in asymptomatic dairy farmers: a study of lymphocytes. *Am Rev Respir Dis.* 1984;139:1046-9.

62. Erkinjuntti-Pekkanen R, Reiman M, Kokkarinen JI. IgG antibodies, chronic bronchitis, and pulmonary function values in farmer's lung patients and matched controls. *Allergy.* 1999;54:1181-7.

63. Sahin H, Brown KK, Curran-Everett D, et al. Chronic hypersensitivity pneumonitis: CT features – comparison with pathologic evidence of fibrosis and survival. *Radiology.* 2007;244:591-8.

64. Silva CI, Churg A, Müller NL. Hypersensitivity pneumonitis: spectrum of high-resolution CT and pathologic findings. *Am J Roentgenol.* 2007;188:334-44.

65. Hansell DM, Wells AV, Padley SP, Müller NL. Hypersensitivity pneumonitis: correlation of individual CT patterns with functional abnormalities. *Radiology.* 1996;199:123-8.

66. Patel RA, Sellami D, Gotway MB, et al. Hypersensitivity pneumonitis: patterns on high-resolution CT. *J Comput Assist Tommogr.* 2000;24:965-70.

67. Hanak V, Golbin JM, Hartman TE, Ryu JH. High-resolution CT findings of parenchymal fibrosis correlate with prognosis in hypersensitivity pneumonitis. *Chest.* 2008;134:133-8.

68. King Jr TE, Tooze JA, Schwarz MI, et al. Predicting survival in idiopathic pulmonary fibrosis: scoring system and survival model. *Am J Respir Crit Care Med.* 2003;168: 1084-90.

69. Cottin V, Densbeck A, Revel D, et al. Nonspecific interstitial pneumonia: individualization of a clinicopathological entity in a series of 12 patients. *Am J Respir Crit Care Med.* 1998;158:1286-93.

70. Veeraraghavan S, Latsi PI, Wells AU, et al. BAL findings in idiopathic nonspecific interstitial pneumonia and usual interstitial pneumonia. *Eur Respir J.* 2003;22:239-44.

71. Barrera L, Mendoza F, Zuniga J, et al. Functional diversity of T-cell subpopulations in subacute and chronic hypersensitivity pneumonitis. *Am J Respir Crit Care Med.* 2008; 177:22-55.

72. Semenzato G. Immunology of interstitial lung diseases: cellular events taking place in the lung of sarcoidosis, hypersensitivity pneumonitis and HIV infection. *Eur Respir J.* 1991;4:94-102.

73. Walker L, Jorres R, Costabel U, Magnussen H. Predictive value of BAL cell differentials in the diagnosis of interstitial lung diseases. *Eur Respir J.* 2004;24:1000-6.

74. Ando M, Konishi K, Yoneda R, Tamura M. Difference in the phenotypes of broncho-alveolar lavage lymphocytes in patients with summer-type hypersensitivity pneumonitis, farmer's lung, ventilation pneumonitis and bird fancier's lung: a report of a nationwide epidemiologic study in Japan. *J Allergy Clin Immunol.* 1991;87:1002-9.

75. Renard S. Th2 cytokine regulation of type I collagen gel contraction mediated by human lung mesenchymal cells. *Am J Physiol.* 2002;282:L1049-56.

76. Sempowski G, Derdak S, Phipps R. Interleukin-4 and interferon-gamma discordantly regulate collagen biosynthesis by functionally distinct lung fibroblast subsets. *J Cell Physiol.* 1996;167:290-6.

77. Semenzato G, Bjermer L, Costabel U, et al. Clinical guidelines and indications for bronchoalveolar lavage (BAL): Report of the European Society of Pneumonology Task Group on BAL: Extrinsic allergic alveolitis. *Eur Respir J.* 1990;3:945-6.

78. Goddard P, Clot J, Jonquet O, et al. Lymphocyte subpopulations in bronchoalveolar lavage of patients with sarcoidosis and hypersensitivity pneumonitis. *Chest.* 1981;80: 447-52.

79. Valenti S, Scordamaglia A, Crimi P, Mereu C. Bronchoalveolar lavage and transbronchial lung biopsy in sarcoidosis and extrinsic allergic alveolitis. *Eur J Respir Dis.* 1982;63: 564-9.

80. Cormier Y, Lacasse Y. Keys to the diagnosis of hypersensitivity pneumonitis: the role of serum precipitins, lung biopsy, and high resolution computed tomography. *Clin Pulm Med.* 1996;3:72-7.

81. American Thoracic Society/European Respiratory Society International Multidisciplinary Consensus Classification of the Idiopathic Interstitial Pneumonias. *Am J Respir Crit Care Med.* 2002;165:277-304.

82. Papanikolaou IC, Drakopanagiotakis F, Polychronopoulas VS. Acute exacerbations of interstitial lung diseases. *Curr Opin Pulm Med.* 2010;16:480-6.

83. Miyazaki Y, Tateishi T, Akashi T, et al. Clinical predictors and histologic appearance of acute exacerbations of chronic hypersensitivity pneumonitis. *Chest.* 2008;134:1265-70.

84. Olson AL, Huie TJ, Groshog SD, et al. Acute exacerbations of fibrotic hypersensitivity pneumonitis: a case series. *Chest.* 2008;134:844-50.

85. Churg A, Wright JL, Tazelaar HD. Acute exacerbations of fibrotic interstitial lung disease. *Histopathology.* 2011;58:525-30.

86. Hyzy R, Huang S, Meyers J, et al. Acute exacerbation of idiopathic pulmonary fibrosis. *Chest.* 2007;132:1652-8.

87. Monkave S, Haahtela T. Farmer's lung—a 5-year follow-up of 86 patients. *Clin Allergy.* 1987;17:143-51.

88. Cormier Y, Belanger J. Long term physiologic outcome after acute farmer's lung. *Chest.* 1985;87:796-800.

89. Bertorelli G, Bocchino V, Olivieri D. Hypersensitivity pneumonitis. In: Interstitial Lung Diseases. Edited by Olivieri D, duBois RM. *Eur Respir Soc Mono.* 2000;14:120-36.

Acute Rejection in the Lung Transplantation Recipient

Timothy PM Whelan

INTRODUCTION

Over 100,000 people die annually in the United States due to chronic lower respiratory disease, and worldwide more than three million people die annually due to chronic obstructive pulmonary disease alone.[1,2] Lung transplantation is a treatment modality available to only a fraction of this population. Yet, it remains an appropriate therapy for the treatment of select patients with advanced lung disease. The first successful lung transplant was performed in 1983 by Cooper and colleagues and since then, has grown from an annual worldwide rate of less than 10 lung transplants per year to nearly 2,708 lung transplants per year in 2007.[3,4] In the last five years, the total volume of lung transplants performed at several centers has increased dramatically, making it more likely that pulmonologists without formal transplant training will be exposed to this patient population. An understanding of the common presentation of acute rejection, the differential diagnosis, and its treatment is vital for the practicing pulmonary physician.

CASE STUDY

A 63-year-old male, status postbilateral lung transplantation six years ago, presented with a two weeks history of increasing cough and sputum production. His symptoms began with the sensation of fevers, but, the patient documented only a temperature of 37.3 °C. The sputum was present mostly in the morning and was clear in color until three days prior to presentation, when it became purulent and more productive. He noted a slight increase in dyspnea walking up a flight of stairs. His wife noted that he has increased respiratory noises when sleeping and, particularly, noted that he was wheezing when in deep sleep. The patient denied orthopnea, paroxysmal nocturnal dyspnea, chest pains, lower extremity edema, lightheadedness, or near syncope. There were no associated gastrointestinal symptoms, and a complete review of systems was otherwise negative.

The patient was currently taking oral cyclosporine 200 mg twice daily. He has been on this dose for approximately eight months without change. His goal cyclosporine level was 150–200 ng/mL and he has been in this range consistently. He denied any new medications. He was taking mycophenolate mofetil 250 mg twice daily. Approximately two months prior to presentation, the MMF was decreased to this dose from 500 mg twice daily due to gastrointestinal side effects; the gastrointestinal symptoms resolved with the decrease in dosage. In addition, the patient continued on his maintenance dose of prednisone 5 mg daily.

His past medical history was significant for a history of severe acute rejection, approximately one year prior to presentation that was treated successfully with high dose corticosteroids and resolved without any further sequelae. His additional medical problems included chronic kidney disease with a baseline creatinine level of 2.5 mg/dL, diabetes mellitus (HbA1c of 6.3), and hypertension that was well controlled with a beta-blocker.

The patient was afebrile with a normal blood pressure and heart rate. Oxygen saturation was 98% on room air with a respiratory rate of 18/minute. He was breathing comfortably at rest. Head, eyes, ears, nose, and throat examination were normal. There was no evidence of lymphadenopathy and lung exam was clear without wheezes, rales, or rhonchi. Cardiac, abdominal, and extremities exams were all normal. Laboratory value of blood and pulmonary function tests are described in tables 8-1 and 8-2. Chest radiograph is shown in figure 8-1.

Table 8-1	Laboratory Values of Blood Investigations
Blood investigations	*Values*
White blood cell count	6.8/μL
Hemoglobin	11.4 g/dL
Platelet count	134,000/μL
INR	1.15
Sodium	144 mEq/L
Potassium	4.4 mEq/L
Chloride	111 mEq/L
Bicarbonate	24 mEq/L
BUN	38 mg/dL
Creatinine	2.6 mg/dL
Glucose	103 mg/dL
Total bilirubin	1.4 mg/dL
Alkaline phosphatase	102 U/L
AST	24 U/L
ALT	22 U/L
Albumin	3.7 g/dL
Cyclosporine level	104 ng/mL

Table 8-2	Spirometry		
	On presentation	Baseline	Percent change
FVC (L)	3.55	3.96	10
FEV$_1$ (L)	2.07	2.52	18
FEV$_1$/FVC (%)	58	64	–

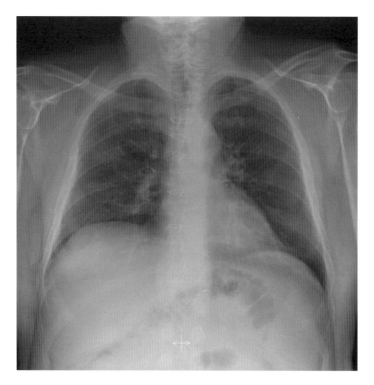

Figure 8-1 Chest radiograph demonstrates status postmedian sternotomy without evidence of focal opacity. In comparison with imaging obtained previously, there is no significant change.

DISCUSSION

The differential diagnosis for the acute onset of dyspnea in the lung transplant recipient is quite broad. Given the known high rates of acute rejection, affecting from 35 to greater than 50% of recipients in the first year after transplant, immunosuppression in this population typically includes a three-drug regimen with a calcinuerin inhibitor, antimetabolite, and prednisone chronically.[4] As a result, clinicians readily include infection versus rejection in their differential.

It is important for the clinician to consider other potential diagnoses in the lung transplant patient who presents with dyspnea.

Deep Venous Thrombosis/Pulmonary Embolism

Multiple reports indicate the elevated prevalence of both deep vein thrombosis (DVT) and pulmonary embolism (PE) in the lung transplant population. Several researchers have identified a prevalence between 8% and 29% depending on identification of a population diagnosed with DVT versus PE.[5-10] Regardless, it is clear these patients are at high risk for DVT, and it should be considered in the differential diagnosis of all patients with dyspnea. Although the risk is greatest in the first-year after transplant, all series have included late occurrences following transplant. Risk factors vary based on the patient population studied and have included increased risk for patients who have a longer length of stay during the first hospitalization, history of cardiopulmonary bypass, older age, diabetes, pneumonia, and idiopathic pulmonary fibrosis.[8,10,11] The cause for the increased risk in the lung transplant recipient is not clear but multiple factors have been suggested including increased de-conditioning of the patients prior to transplant as well as prolonged and continued inflammation following transplant.

Acute Coronary Syndrome

There is a paucity of data on the incidence and prevalence of significant ischemic heart disease after lung transplantation. This is likely due to the low incidence of transplanting patients with known significant coronary artery disease. In the early years of lung transplantation, potential candidates with coronary artery disease were most likely excluded from listing. More recently, dogmatic decision making related to risks associated with pre-existing coronary artery disease appears to be softening. Investigators have documented that patients with mild to moderate coronary artery disease (CAD) (stenosis < 50%) do well after transplant.[12] In addition, it has been shown that cardiac surgery in conjunction with the lung transplant procedure can be performed safely.[13-16] Further affirming these findings, the current consensus guidelines for referral and listing for lung transplantation list coronary artery disease as a relative contraindication.[17]

Other factors that will likely impact on the risk of development of ischemic cardiac disease after lung transplant include the trend to transplant older patients[4] and, in the United States, more frequently transplant patients with idiopathic pulmonary fibrosis.[18] It has been shown that patients with idiopathic pulmonary fibrosis have a higher baseline risk of coronary artery disease than patients with chronic obstructive pulmonary disease.[19-21] The mechanisms that result in this increased preoperative risk may not be affected by transplantation. This could mean an increased risk in the postoperative population as well.

In addition to the increasing likelihood of modern era transplant recipients having some element of coronary artery disease at the time of their transplant surgery, common comorbidities after transplant increase the risk for development of coronary artery disease. These include high rates of hypertension, chronic kidney disease, and hypercholesterolemia.[4] The end result is that ischemic heart disease remains on the differential when evaluating patients for new onset dyspnea. A low threshold to evaluate these patients with routine ECG and subsequent functional testing is appropriate.

Chronic Kidney Disease (CKD)

Volume overload as well as dyspnea related to acid-base disorders secondary to chronic kidney disease should also be included in the differential diagnosis. Lung transplant recipients have a high-risk of developing CKD with nearly 70% of recipients having either CKD stage III (GFR 30–59 mL/min/1.73 m^2) or stage IV (GFR 15–29 mL/min/1.73 m^2) at one year following lung transplant.[22] The major inciting event related to this risk is the need to use calcineurin inhibitor-based immunosuppression to prevent the development of acute rejection after lung transplantation. As this class of medications is routinely used after lung transplantation, additional risk factors have been identified that further increase the probability of development of CKD. These risk factors include older age and a history of acute kidney dysfunction in the first month after transplantation. As the lung transplant recipient population is increasing in age, careful evaluation of volume status and the potential impact this may have on the development of dyspnea is appropriate.

Pulmonary Infections

A full discussion of the potential pulmonary pathogens that the immuno-compromised host is at risk to develop is beyond the scope of this manuscript. However, it is worthwhile mentioning some key issues that are particular to the lung transplant recipient. Similar to immunocompetent patients, the lung transplant recipient is at risk to develop usual community-acquired pathogens. Community respiratory viruses deserve special mention, as they are extremely common in the lung transplant recipient.[23,24] Several series have documented the association of paramyxoviruses (i.e., respiratory syncytial virus, human metapneumovirus) with poor outcomes acutely.[25,26] Viral infections have also been implicated in the development of bronchiolitis obliterans syndrome (BOS).[27,28] Bronchiolitis obliterans syndrome, chronic lung allograft dysfunction, or chronic rejection are common terms referring to the development of fibroproliferative small airways disease that is evident clinically by obstruction on pulmonary function testing. This complication after lung transplantation is the leading cause of late mortality.[4] Although treatment options are limited for respiratory viral infections, given their association with poor outcomes acutely and their association with long-term pulmonary complications, consideration of early intervention is appropriate. Several studies demonstrate that an early intervention strategy may improve outcomes.[29-31]

In addition, to typical community respiratory pathogens, consideration of the patient's past history should be given. Given the high rates of hospitalization (particularly in the first-year after transplantation),[4] consideration of hospital acquired infections is appropriate. Furthermore, a history of BOS predisposes patients to colonization with Gram-negative organisms (i.e., *Pseudomonas*) and pathogenic fungi.

Community-acquired pathogens, including viral infections, as well as the individual patient's risk for associated colonization with antibiotic resistant organisms must be considered when selecting empiric antibiotic coverage for the acutely ill lung transplant recipient.

Acute Rejection

Acute rejection remains one of the most common complications early after lung transplantation. It is consistently reported in the literature to occur in over 50% of lung transplant recipients in the first year following lung transplantation.[4,32,33] Acute rejection is a T cell mediated response to nonself antigens. These antigens include the human leukocyte antigens (HLA) but other non-HLA antigens can also fuel the response. Histologically, acute rejection is characterized by perivascular and subendothelial mononuclear infiltrates and by lymphocytic bronchitis and bronchiolitis.

Interleukin-2 (IL-2) is integral to the development of acute rejection. It is for this reason that calcineurin inhibitors are the backbone of immunosuppression regimens in transplantation. Goal drug levels are set by the primary lung transplant center and are based on the balance between the development of acute rejection and toxicities associated with the medications. When the patient presented, he recently decreased the dosage of mycophenolate mofetil which may increase his risk of acute rejection. Also, the patient had a cyclosporine level that was significantly lower than his goal level. He had not had a change in dosage in several months. It is extremely important to ask patients about concomitant medications as the calcineurin inhibitors are metabolized via CYP3A4, and there are many potential drug-drug interactions that can either increase or decrease these levels (Table 8-3).

Table 8-3 Common Drug-drug Interactions Involving Calcineurin Inhibitors	
Increase calcineurin inhibitor levels	*Decrease calcineurin inhibitor levels*
Azole antifungals	Rifampin
Diltiazem	Phenobarbital
Macrolide antibiotics	Phenytoin

Milder episodes of acute rejection can lack respiratory symptoms or be entirely asymptomatic. With higher levels of acute rejection, typical complaints are similar to acute respiratory infection with cough, fever, malaise, dyspnea, and/or decreased oxygen saturation. Treatment of acute rejection requires significantly augmenting the individual's immunosuppression. Given the similarity in symptoms to infection and the opposite therapeutic aims, infection must be excluded as a potential etiology.

Noninvasive testing (PFTs, radiographic imaging, serum blood work, sputum culture) is helpful in the management of these patients; however, noninvasive testing is neither sensitive nor specific for identifying patients with acute lung rejection. Pulmonary function testing has consistently been shown to be an effective tool for serially following patients.[34] During an episode of acute rejection, the forced expiratory volume in one second (FEV_1) will decline. Transplant centers typically consider a reduction in FEV_1 of 10% from baseline as significant. Unfortunately, this is not specific for acute rejection and can only be used as supportive evidence to consider further investigation.

Additionally, chest radiographs appear to be more sensitive in the first several weeks after transplant surgery and then can be completely normal despite evidence of acute rejection on transbronchial biopsy.[35-37] Computed tomography machines are ubiquitous in the community and, as such, high resolution computed tomography use is more frequent. There is not a wealth of data on CT imaging and its correlation with the diagnosis of acute rejection; however, evidence of ground glass opacities on CT imaging warrants evaluation and these findings may help direct the pulmonologist to the best area for bronchoalveolar lavage and transbronchial biopsies.[38,39] Similar to chest radiographs, normal chest tomography cannot absolutely exclude acute rejection.

Bronchoscopy with bronchoalveolar lavage and transbronchial biopsies remains the gold standard for identifying acute rejection. Multiple investigators have identified correlations of findings in BAL fluid with acute rejection; however, these associations are not currently specific enough to obviate the need for histological confirmation.[40-42] It is also important to note here that the histologic findings consistent with acute rejection can be seen with viral infection and *Pneumocystis jeroveci pneumonia*. The BAL provides excellent sensitivity and specificity for the identification of an underlying infection. As a result, BAL is an integral part of the evaluation of the patient considered to have acute rejection. It essentially excludes infection as the cause of the patient's complaints. Multiple BAL studies are typically sent as outlined in table 8-4.

Transbronchial biopsies have demonstrated very high rates of sensitivity in animal models when adequate tissue is obtained.[43] The lung rejection study group consensus was that at least five pieces of alveolated tissue, each containing

Table 8-4	Useful Studies from BAL to Determine Infection versus Rejection
Cell count with differential	Viral culture
Gram's stain	Cytomegalovirus PCR
Quantitative bacterial culture	Respiratory viral PCR panel
Fungal culture	Cytological examination for: *Pneumocystis*,
Acid-fast bacillus culture and stain	malignancy, viral inclusions, fungal elements
Nocardia culture	

bronchioles and more than 100 air sacs are necessary to grade acute rejection confidently.[44] Typically, the bronchoscopist must obtain at least twice this number of transbronchial biopsy specimens to achieve this volume of tissue.[33] Grading of the specimens is based on the extent of mononuclear infiltrates noted (Table 8-5). Evaluation of histologic grading by community pathologists has never been formally studied. Transplant centers have demonstrated good intra/interobserver agreement amongst experienced pathologists, although there is conflicting data.[45,46] The discrepancy amongst readings is accentuated when the pathologist must determine the appropriate grading of acute rejection within the specimen. It is advisable that transbronchial biopsy specimens be reviewed by an experienced pathologist familiar with the classification system for grading acute rejection.

Table 8-5	Histologic Grading of Acute Rejection
Grade	*Description of histologic findings*
A0 (normal or no rejection)	Normal parenchyma
A1 (minimal acute rejection)	Infrequent perivascular mononuclear infiltrates; venules are cuffed by lymphocytes forming a ring of two or three cells in thickness
A2 (mild acute rejection)	More frequent perivascular mononuclear infiltrates affecting venules and arterioles and recognizeable at low power. Endothialitis may be present. There is no obvious infiltration by mononuclear cells in the adjacent alveolar septa or air spaces
A3 (moderate acute rejection)	Readily recognizable cuffing of venules and arterioles by dense perivascular mononuclear infiltrates; extension into into perivascular and peribronchiolar alveolar septae and air spaces
A4 (severe acute rejection)	Diffuse perivascular, interstitial, and air space infiltrates; prominent alveolar pneumocyte damage and endothialitis; may have intra-alveolar necrosis, hyaline membranes, hemorrhage, neutrophils

Adapted from Stewart et al. Revision of the 1996 working formulation for the standardization of nomenclature in the diagnosis of lung rejection. *J Heart Lung Transplant.* 2007;26:1229-42.

MANAGEMENT OF CASE STUDY

Bronchoscopy with bronchoalveolar lavage was performed. Gram's stain and cytologic examination were negative as were all cultures and screening for respiratory virus. Fourteen transbronchial biopsies were obtained, and these provided adequate tissue to demonstrate grade A2 rejection.

15 mg/kg of intravenous methylprednisolone was administered each day for three days. The patient's symptoms improved significantly on day 2, and by day 4, the patient complained of mild fatigue; but cough, sputum production, and dyspnea were completely resolved. This is a typical course for acute rejection; it responds quickly to high dose corticosteroid therapy.[47] The patient was then placed on a brief prednisone burst (1 mg/kg) and tapered back to his baseline dosing over the next 10 days.[48] As this patient had a history of exposure to cytomegalovirus (CMV-IgG positive) and is at risk for reactivation, he was also placed on oral valgancyclovir prophylaxis for the next four weeks.

Follow-up of the patient after treatment remains extremely important. Multiple episodes of acute rejection are strongly associated with the development of bronchiolitis obliterans syndrome. It is known that some patients treated for acute rejection will continue to show persistent declines in their FEV_1 despite appropriate therapy. In addition, some patients will have evidence of persistent acute rejection on histology after treatment with apparent resolution of symptoms.[49] For these reasons, the lung transplant recipient diagnosed with acute rejection should have close follow-up after treatment with symptom assessment, pulmonary function testing, and consideration of repeat bronchoscopy with transbronchial biopsies. For patients who continue to show evidence of declines and/or persistent acute rejection, discussion with the primary transplant center for further treatment options is appropriate.

REFERENCES

1. Fast Stats. Deaths and Mortality in the US [Internet]: Center for Disease Control and Prevention; c2010 [cited 2010 08/31]. Available from: http://www.cdc.gov/nchs/fastats/deaths.htm.
2. Mathers C, Fat DM, Boerma JT. World Health Organization. The global burden of disease: 2004 update. Geneva, Switzerland: World Health Organization; 2008. The 2004 update of the Global burden of disease was primarily carried out by Colin Mathers and Doris Ma Fat, in collaboration with other WHO staff, WHO technical program and UNAIDS. The report was written by Colin Mathers, Ties Boerma and Doris Ma Fat.
3. Unilateral lung transplantation for pulmonary fibrosis. Toronto Lung Transplant Group. *N Engl J Med.* 1986;314:1140-5.
4. Christie JD, Edwards LB, Aurora P, et al. The registry of the international society for heart and lung transplantation: twenty-sixth official adult lung and heart-lung transplantation report-2009. *J Heart Lung Transplant.* 2009;10:1031-49.

5. Burns KE, Iacono AT. Pulmonary embolism on postmortem examination: an under-recognized complication in lung-transplant recipients? *Transplantation.* 2004;77:692-8.

6. Burns KE, Iacono AT. Incidence of clinically unsuspected pulmonary embolism in mechanically ventilated lung transplant recipients. *Transplantation.* 2003;76:964-8.

7. Izbicki G, Bairey O, Shitrit D, Lahav J, Kramer MR. Increased thromboembolic events after lung transplantation. *Chest.* 2006;129:412-6.

8. Kahan ES, Petersen G, Gaughan JP, Criner GJ. High incidence of venous thromboembolic events in lung transplant recipients. *J Heart Lung Transplant.* 2007;26:339-44.

9. Kroshus TJ, Kshettry VR, Hertz MI, Bolman RM, 3rd. Deep venous thrombosis and pulmonary embolism after lung transplantation. *J Thorac Cardiovasc Surg.* 1995;110:540-4.

10. Nathan SD, Barnett SD, Urban BA, Nowalk C, Moran BR, Burton N. Pulmonary embolism in idiopathic pulmonary fibrosis transplant recipients. *Chest.* 2003;123:1758-63.

11. Yegen HA, Lederer DJ, Barr RG, et al. Risk factors for venous thromboembolism after lung transplantation. *Chest.* 2007;132:547-53.

12. Choong CK, Meyers BF, Guthrie TJ, Trulock EP, Patterson GA, Moazami N. Does the presence of preoperative mild or moderate coronary artery disease affect the outcomes of lung transplantation? *Ann Thorac Surg.* 2006;82:1038-42.

13. Parekh K, Meyers BF, Patterson GA, Guthrie TJ, Trulock EP, Damiano RJ Jr, Moazami N. Outcome of lung transplantation for patients requiring concomitant cardiac surgery. *J Thorac Cardiovasc Surg.* 2005;130:859-63.

14. Patel VS, Palmer SM, Messier RH, Davis RD. Clinical outcome after coronary artery revascularization and lung transplantation. *Ann Thorac Surg.* 2003;75:372-7.

15. Khatchatourian G, Chevalley C, Spiliopoulos A, Licker M. Myocardial revascularization and bilateral lung transplantation without cardiopulmonary bypass. *Eur J Cardiothorac Surg.* 2001;20:1042-4.

16. Lee JS, Brown KK, Cool C, Lynch DA. Diffuse pulmonary neuroendocrine cell hyperplasia: radiologic and clinical features. *J Comput Assist Tomogr.* 2002;26:180-4.

17. Orens JB, Estenne M, Arcasoy S, et al. Pulmonary Scientific Council of the International Society for Heart and Lung Transplantation. International guidelines for the selection of lung transplant candidates: 2006 update--a consensus report from the pulmonary scientific council of the international society for heart and lung transplantation. *J Heart Lung Transplant.* 2006;25:745-55.

18. Scientific Registry of Transplant Recipients: Transplant Recipient Characteristics, Deceased Donor Transplants Patients Transplanted between 1/1/2009 and 12/31/2009 National Report for Lung [Internet] [cited 2010]. Available from: http://www.ustransplant.org/csr/current/nationalViewer.aspx?o=LU&t=07C.

19. Nathan SD, Basavaraj A, Reichner C, et al. Prevalence and impact of coronary artery disease in idiopathic pulmonary fibrosis. *Respir Med.* 2010;104:1035-41.

20. Izbicki G, Ben-Dor I, Shitrit D, Bendayan D, Aldrich TK, Kornowski R, Kramer MR. The prevalence of coronary artery disease in end-stage pulmonary disease: is pulmonary fibrosis a risk factor? *Respir Med.* 2009;103:1346-9.

21. Kizer JR, Zisman DA, Blumenthal NP, Kotloff RM, Kimmel SE, Strieter RM, Arcasoy SM, Ferrari VA, Hansen-Flaschen J. Association between pulmonary fibrosis and coronary artery disease. *Arch Intern Med.* 2004;164:551-6.

22. Canales M, Youssef P, Spong R, Ishani A, Savik K, Hertz M, Ibrahim HN. Predictors of chronic kidney disease in long-term survivors of lung and heart-lung transplantation. *Am J Transplant.* 2006;6:2157-63.

23. Weinberg A, Zamora MR, Li S, Torres F, Hodges TN. The value of polymerase chain reaction for the diagnosis of viral respiratory tract infections in lung transplant recipients. *J Clin Virol.* 2002;25:171-5.

24. Kumar D, Husain S, Chen MH, et al. A prospective molecular surveillance study evaluating the clinical impact of community-acquired respiratory viruses in lung transplant recipients. *Transplantation.* 2010;89:1028-33.

25. Hopkins P, McNeil K, Kermeen F, Musk M, McQueen E, Mackay I, Sloots T, Nissen M. Human metapneumovirus in lung transplant recipients and comparison to respiratory syncytial virus. *Am J Respir Crit Care Med.* 2008;178:876-81.

26. McCurdy LH, Milstone A, Dummer S. Clinical features and outcomes of paramyxoviral infection in lung transplant recipients treated with ribavirin. *J Heart Lung Transplant.* 2003;22:745-53.

27. Billings JL, Hertz MI, Savik K, Wendt CH. Respiratory viruses and chronic rejection in lung transplant recipients. *J Heart Lung Transplant.* 2002;21:559-66.

28. Khalifah AP, Hachem RR, Chakinala MM, et al. Respiratory viral infections are a distinct risk for bronchiolitis obliterans syndrome and death. *Am J Respir Crit Care Med.* 2004;170:181-7.

29. Weill D. Donor criteria in lung transplantation: an issue revisited. *Chest.* 2002;121: 2029-31.

30. Sparrelid E, Ljungman P, Ekelof-Andstrom E, et al. Ribavirin therapy in bone marrow transplant recipients with viral respiratory tract infections. *Bone Marrow Transplant.* 1997;19:905-8.

31. Tsitsikas DA, Oakervee H, Cavenagh JD, Gribben J, Agrawal SG, Mattes FM. Treatment of respiratory syncytial virus infection in hemopoietic stem cell transplant recipients with aerosolized ribavirin and the humanized monoclonal antibody palivizumab: a single centre experience. *Br J Haematol.* 2009;146:574-6.

32. Zuckermann A, Reichenspurner H, Birsan T, Treede H, Deviatko E, Reichart B, Klepetko W. Cyclosporine A versus tacrolimus in combination with mycophenolate mofetil and steroids as primary immunosuppression after lung transplantation: one-year results of a 2-center prospective randomized trial. *J Thorac Cardiovasc Surg.* 2003;125:891-900.

33. Hopkins PM, Aboyoun CL, Chhajed PN, Malouf MA, Plit ML, Rainer SP, Glanville AR. Prospective analysis of 1,235 transbronchial lung biopsies in lung transplant recipients. *J Heart Lung Transplant.* 2002;21:1062-7.

34. Van Muylem A, Melot C, Antoine M, Knoop C, Estenne M. Role of pulmonary function in the detection of allograft dysfunction after heart-lung transplantation. *Thorax.* 1997; 52:643-7.

35. Bergin CJ, Castellino RA, Blank N, Berry GJ, Sibley RK, Starnes VA. Acute lung rejection after heart-lung transplantation: correlation of findings on chest radiographs with lung biopsy results. *Am J Roentgenol.* 1990;155:23-7.

36. Kundu S, Herman SJ, Larhs A, Rappaport DC, Weisbrod GL, Maurer J, Chamberlain D, Winton T. Correlation of chest radiographic findings with biopsy-proven acute lung rejection. *J Thorac Imaging.* 1999;14:178-84.

37. Millet B, Higenbottam TW, Flower CD, Stewart S, Wallwork J. The radiographic appearances of infection and acute rejection of the lung after heart-lung transplantation. *Am Rev Respir Dis.* 1989;140:62-7.

38. Loubeyre P, Revel D, Delignette A, Loire R, Mornex JF. High-resolution computed tomographic findings associated with histologically diagnosed acute lung rejection in heart-lung transplant recipients. *Chest.* 1995;107:132-8.

39. Herber S, Lill J, Heussel CP, Mayer E, Thelen M, Kauczor HU. Acute or chronic transplant rejection—high resolution CT of the chest in lung transplant recipients. *Rofo.* 2001;173:822-9.

40. Patil J, Lande JD, Li N, Berryman TR, King RA, Hertz MI. Bronchoalveolar lavage cell gene expression in acute lung rejection: development of a diagnostic classifier. *Transplantation.* 2008;85:224-31.

41. Bhorade SM, Yu A, Vigneswaran WT, Alex CG, Garrity ER. Elevation of interleukin-15 protein expression in bronchoalveolar fluid in acute lung allograft rejection. *Chest.* 2007;131:533-8.

42. Vanaudenaerde BM, Dupont LJ, Wuyts WA, et al. The role of interleukin-17 during acute rejection after lung transplantation. *Eur Respir J.* 2006;27:779-87.

43. Tazelaar HD, Nilsson FN, Rinaldi M, Murtaugh P, McDougall JC, McGregor CG. The sensitivity of transbronchial biopsy for the diagnosis of acute lung rejection. *J Thorac Cardiovasc Surg.* 1993;105:674-8.

44. Yousem SA, Berry GJ, Cagle PT, et al. Revision of the 1990 working formulation for the classification of pulmonary allograft rejection: lung rejection study group. *J Heart Lung Transplant.* 1996;15:1-15.

45. Chakinala MM, Ritter J, Gage BF, Aloush AA, Hachem RH, Lynch JP, Patterson GA, Trulock EP. Reliability for grading acute rejection and airway inflammation after lung transplantation. *J Heart Lung Transplant.* 2005;24:652-7.

46. Stephenson A, Flint J, English J, Vedal S, Fradet G, Chittock D, Levy RD. Interpretation of transbronchial lung biopsies from lung transplant recipients: inter- and intraobserver agreement. *Can Respir J.* 2005;12:75-7.

47. Sibley RK, Berry GJ, Tazelaar HD, Kraemer MR, Theodore J, Marshall SE, Billingham ME, Starnes VA. The role of transbronchial biopsies in the management of lung transplant recipients. *J Heart Lung Transplant.* 1993;12:308-24.

48. Hertz MI, Bolman RM, University of Minnesota. Physicians Transplant Program, Fairview Health Services. In: Marshall I Hertz, RM Bolman III, et al (Eds); *Manual of Lung Transplant Medical Care.* 2nd ed. Minneapolis: Fairview Publications; 2001. Transplant Services, a unique partnership of University of Minnesota Physicians Transplant Program and Fairview Health Services.

49. Whelan TP, Hertz MI. Allograft rejection after lung transplantation. *Clin Chest Med.* 2005;26:599-612, vi.

Drug-induced Respiratory Disease

J Terrill Huggins

INTRODUCTION

Since Sir William Osler described the effects of morphine in eliciting pulmonary edema in 1880s, the number of drugs causing lung toxicity now exceeds by 500 with more than 50 distinctive patterns of respiratory involvement. Drug-induced lung injury (DILI) may involve the airways, lung parenchyma, mediastinum, pleura, pulmonary vasculature, and the neuromuscular system.[1,2] Some drugs mimic well-described clinical syndromes with isolated pulmonary toxicity such as acute respiratory distress syndrome (ARDS); however, multisystem presentations can occur in the setting of drug-induced vasculitis. DILI is often a diagnosis of exclusion because there are no specific clinical, laboratory, radiographic, or histologic features that firmly establish the diagnosis. It is often unpredictable, presenting challenges to both diagnosis and management. It is imperative for the clinician to have a high clinical suspicion for drug-related causes in patients who are present with respiratory system abnormalities.

Management of DILI includes drug withdrawal, supportive care and at times, corticosteroids, depending on its clinical presentation. This chapter will discuss the common clinical, radiographic, and histological patterns of lung injury, discuss diagnosis and treatment, and details of the pulmonary toxicity of emerging biological agents, antineoplastics, and commonly encountered medications.

EPIDEMIOLOGY AND MECHANISMS OF PULMONARY TOXICITY

The first extensive review of DILI was written by Rosenow in the early 1970s and included 30 medications.[1] Since then, the number of drugs implicated in DILI is in the hundreds. The true frequency is unknown for most of the drugs and limited case reports exist for medications implicated in causing toxicity. Furthermore, it is problematic to ascertain drug causality, when a pulmonary toxicity pattern attributed to the drug can also occur as a consequence of the underlying disease.

An excellent up-to-date and web-based resource is pneumotox.com.[2] This website lists all the drugs implicated in lung injury, reports the frequency of toxicity, and provides the references for further reading. It is clear that drugs are important contributors to lung toxicity. Medications which are most commonly implicated include amiodarone, transfusion of plasma containing blood products, methotrexate, numerous chemotherapeutics, biological agents, such as anti-TNF alfa, angiotensin-converting enzyme inhibitors (ACEI), and nonsteroidal anti-inflammatory drugs (NSAIDs).

At risk patients for DILI typically are older, have underlying inflammatory conditions such as rheumatoid arthritis, and are receiving concurrent toxic agents, such as chemotherapy and radiation. In patients with rheumatoid arthritis, the risk of developing acute methotrexate pneumonitis ranges from 0.3 to 11.6%.[3-6] Drug administration most commonly described in DILI usually involves oral and parenteral routes; however, inhalational and intrathecal administration has been implicated.[3] Synergistic effects may occur when multiple agents, with known risk for pulmonary toxicity, are administered together. This often occurs when multiple chemotherapeutic drugs are coadministered or given concurrently with thoracic radiation. Toxicity may be dose-related, as carmustine, bleomycin, paclitaxel, and amiodarone result in pulmonary toxicity.[3]

Radiation recall pneumonitis is a phenomenon which occurs in patients who receive prior radiation and are also exposed to antineoplastic agents. Shortly after the initiation of the chemotherapy, an acute presentation of fever, cough, dyspnea, and hypoxia develops. Diffuse pulmonary infiltrates are seen on chest imaging. It is believed that prior radiation may cause subclinical parenchymal injury, which may have an additive effect when another pulmonary insult occurs. Radiation-induced injury to the type II pneumocytes reducing the reparative mechanisms of the lung and hypersensitivity reactions; both are plausible mechanisms for the development of radiation recall pneumonitis.[4] Antineoplastic agents associated with radiation recall pneumonitis are listed in table 9-1.

Mostly, drugs do not cause direct cell toxicity and some biotransformation is required. Initially, drugs undergo oxidative reactions mediated by the cytochrome P-450 superfamily of enzymes during phase-I biotransformation. Phase-II reactions occur and consist of conjugate reactions, whereby metabolites are coupled to yield more water soluble compounds for elimination.[7] The process of biotransformation

Table 9-1	Chemotherapeutic Agents Most Likely Related to Radiation Recall Pneumonitis	
Adriamycin	Gefitinib
Carmustine (BCNU)	Gemcitabine
Doxorubicin	Paclitaxel
Etoposide	Trastuzumab

may produce chemical structures which have increased cell cytotoxicity. Most reactive metabolites result from phase-I reactions, and if these reactive metabolites are not readily removed by enzymatic or nonenzymatic reactions, they may cause cell injury, resulting in tissue toxicity.

Production of activated oxygen species occurs during bioactivation of drugs. Reactive electrophilic metabolites bind covalently with essential cellular macromolecules or nucleic acids resulting in cell dysfunction.[7] Indirect or direct cytotoxicity to the lung may result from this mechanism. On the other hand, a hypersensitivity or allergic mechanism may be responsible for drug-induced lung toxicity. Evidence for this mechanism may only be circumstantial and supported by the presence of eosinophils in lung lavage or serum; specific antibodies are rarely documented.

In contrast, a model of drug-induced immunologic injury, where the drug acts as an immunostimulant to induce monoclonal expansion of lymphocytes, exists for some cases of drug-induced lupus (DIL). Penicillamine has been shown to induce a Goodpasture's reaction. In addition, antineutrophil cytoplasmic antibody (ANCA)-positive angiitis, with or without capillaritis, has been described with propylthiouracil, minocycline, sulfasalazine, and allopurinol.

An additional mechanism accounting for a substantial number of drug-related cases of pulmonary toxicity occurs in unpredictable circumstances often following minimal and small amounts of drug exposure. In this scenario, the mechanism of metabolic idiosyncrasy is responsible. Metabolic idiosyncrasy implies host intolerance which is genetically determined.[7] Therefore, in a susceptible host, the metabolic idiosyncrasy mechanism could result from an inability to adequately biotransform the drug or cope with active metabolites; the host develops an immunologically acquired intolerance that is not related to prior drug exposure. Toxicity susceptibility, which is not based on an idiosyncratic mechanism includes the underlying disease for which the drug is being prescribed; the presence of liver or renal failure; and the impact of concomitant drugs utilizing the same enzymatic pathways and altering the pharmacokinetics of the offending drugs.[7]

PATHOLOGIC AND RADIOGRAPHIC FINDINGS OF DRUG-INDUCED LUNG DISEASE

Histopathological patterns associated with pulmonary drug reactions are highly variable. These patterns include pulmonary edema, diffuse alveolar damage (DAD), alveolar proteinosis-like reaction, alveolar hemorrhage, organizing pneumonia, usual interstitial pneumonia (UIP), diffuse cellular infiltrates with or without granulomas, nonspecific interstitial pneumonia (NSIP), lymphocytic interstitial pneumonia (LIP), acute or chronic eosinophilic pneumonia, small vessel angiitis, bronchiolitis obliterans with organizing pneumonia (BOOP), bronchiolitis obliterans (BO), pulmonary arterial hypertension (PAH), and pulmonary veno-occlusive disease.[8,9]

Nonspecific Interstitial Pneumonia

It is evident that all forms of interstitial pneumonitis can be associated with drug therapy, but the most common pattern is NSIP.[8,10] High-resolution chest tomography (HRCT) findings of NSIP pattern most often show patchy ground-glass opacities or consolidation with reticular changes, which has a peripheral and basilar predominance. Honeycombing is uncommon in NSIP.[10-16] Drug-induced NSIP most commonly occurs with amiodarone, methotrexate, carmustine, gold salts, and nitrofurantoin. High-attenuation areas in the lung parenchyma seen on HRCT are characteristic findings of amiodarone lung toxicity. Upper lobe predominance is seen with carmustine.[16]

Usual Interstitial Pneumonia

In cases of drug-related UIP, chemotherapeutics are most commonly implicated, especially bleomycin and methotrexate. The UIP pattern on HRCT shows subpleural honeycombing, which appears as cystic airspaces with thick walls. Fibrosis leads to traction bronchiectasis and bronchiolectasis.[8,17-19] The presence of prominent honeycombing, with subpleural and basilar predominance on HRCT, is diagnostic of UIP pattern.

Hypersensitivity Pneumonitis

Methotrexate, bleomycin, cyclophosphamide, nitrofurantoin, penicillamine, non-steroidal anti-inflammatory drugs, and sulfonamides have been implicated in hypersensitivity reaction. Chest radiographs may show subtle areas of nonspecific opacities or small areas of consolidation. On HRCT, bilateral, patchy, ground-glass opacities are seen. Air-trapping on expiratory imaging with ground-glass centrilobular nodules is a more classic finding on HRCT for hypersensitivity pneumonitis.[19-22]

Desquamative Interstitial Pneumonia

Drug-related cases of DIP have been reported. Drugs most commonly implicated include nitrofurantoin, busulfan, and sulfasalazine.[2] Rare DIP reactions have been described with interferon-alfa, rituximab, and sirolimus.[2,23] The clinical presentation is typically chronic progressive dyspnea (Table 9-2). The predominant finding on HRCT is the presence of ground-glass attenuation that involves the middle and lower lung zones with a peripheral distribution. Irregular lines of attenuation,

Table 9-2	Drug-induced Desquamative Intersitial Pneumonia
Common	**Rare**
Nitrofurantoin	Interferon-alfa
Busulfan	Rituximab
Sulfasalazine	Sirolimus

suggestive of fibrosis, may be seen in half of the cases, with cystic changes in a third. The radiographic distribution of DIP is similar to that seen in UIP; however, the greater extent of ground-glass attenuation and the paucity of cystic changes in DIP should enable distinction from UIP.[24] The main pathological findings in DIP are homogeneous distribution of macrophages in the airspaces, a mild-to-moderate interstitial chronic inflammation, minimal fibrosis, and epithelial cell metaplasia.

LIP and Pulmonary Alveolar Proteinosis

Drug-induced LIP and pulmonary alveolar proteinosis (PAP) represent a rare form of DILI. To date, only two drugs, captopril and phenytoin, have been described causing a LIP reaction.[25,26] In these instances, drug discontinuation resulted in resolution of symptoms. Currently, three drugs (mitomycin-C, leflunomide, and sirolimus) have been implicated in causing PAP. The strongest association of drug-induced pulmonary alveolar proteinosis has been described with mitomycin-C[2] (Table 9-3). Recent reports of PAP have been associated with the immunosuppressant, sirolimus, in transplant patients. PAP is a progressive lung disease, characterized by the accumulation of surfactant-like material in the lungs, leading to decreased pulmonary function with shortness of breath and cough as common symptoms. Discontinuation of sirolimus and initiation of tacrolimus led to resolution of PAP without recurrence of hemolytic-uremic syndrome (HUS) in this case report.[27]

Bronchiolitis Obliterans

Bronchiolitis obliterans has been described as following gold salts, penicillamine, sulfasalazine, and busulfan.[28,29] Drug-induced BO is controversial with the use of penicillamine and sulfasalazine since the underlying diseases, for which these two drugs are used, rheumatoid arthritis and inflammatory bowel disease are also BO-causative. Hyperinflation, with decreased peripheral vascular markings, is often detected on chest radiographs. HRCT findings include hyperinflation, bronchial wall thickening, mosaic perfusion, and air trapping on expiratory imaging.[29-31] Fibrosis with obliteration of the terminal respiratory bronchioles is seen histologically.

Bronchiolitis Obliterans with Organizing Pneumonia

Numerous drugs can result in a drug-induced BOOP pattern. Common offenders include amiodarone, gold salts, bleomycin, carbamazepine, cyclophosphamide, ergot derivatives, hexamethonium, minocycline, nilatamide, nitrofurantoin, phenytoin,

Table 9-3	Drug-induced Pulmonary Alveolar Proteinosis
Mitomycin-C*	Sirolimus
Leflunomide	

*Strongest association of pulmonary alveolar proteinosis is described with mitomycin-C.

and penicillamine[2] (Table 9-4). Focal involvement, mimicking pulmonary masses, has also been described with amiodarone. However, most of the cases of drug-induced BOOP involve the lungs diffusely.[32] Typical radiographic findings include patchy, bilateral alveolar infiltrates, or ground-glass opacities which have a peripheral predominance. A peribronchovascular distribution and nodular consolidation have also been described.[33,34] The morphological pattern of BOOP consists of fibromyxoid connective tissue plugs that fill distal airspaces and respiratory bronchioles.

Table 9-4 Drug-induced Bronchiolitis Obliterans Organizing Pneumonia	
Drugs	*Strength of association*
Amiodarone	+ + +
Bleomycin	+ + +
Cyclophosphamide	+ + +
Carbamazepine	+ + +
Ergot derivatives	+ + +
Gold salts	+ + +
Hexamethonium	+ + +
Minocycline	+ + +
Nilutamide	+ + +
Nitrofurantoin	+ + +
Penicillamine	+ + +
Phenytoin	+ + +
Radiation	+ + +
Acebutolol	+ +
Amphotericin B	+ +
Doxorubicin	+ +
Dihydroergocryptine	+ +
Hydralazine	+ +
Interferon-alfa	+ +
Interferon-beta	+ +
Mecamylamine	+ +
Mesalamine	+ +
Rituximab	+ +
Simvastatin	+ +
Trastuzumab	+ +
Abacavir	+
Azathioprine	+

Continued

Continued

Drugs	Strength of association
Barbiturates	+
Betaxolol	+
Busulfan	+
Chlorambucil	+
Cephalosporins	+
Clomipramine	+
Dihydroergotamine	+
Everolimus	+
Heroin	+
Lenalidomide	+
Loxoprofen	+
Methotrexate	+
Mitomycin-C	+
Pravastatin	+
Risedronate	+
Sotalol	+
Sulindac	+
Tacrolimus	+
Temozolomide	+
Thalidomide	+
Ticlopidine	+
Topotecan	+

+ + + denotes drugs with frequent association; + + denotes drugs with occasional association; and + denotes drugs with rare association.

Noncardiogenic Pulmonary Edema with or without Diffuse Alveolar Damage

Noncardiogenic pulmonary edema and ARDS are common clinical manifestations of drug-induced lung diseases. The list of drugs that cause pulmonary edema and ARDS is extensive. Approximately 90 drugs have been implicated as a cause of pulmonary edema (Table 9-5) and 30 drugs have been reported as a cause of ARDS (Table 9-6). Drugs which are most commonly implicated in causing diffuse alveolar damage include transfusion of plasma containing blood products, amiodarone, cyclophosphamide, bleomycin, carmustine, mitomycin-C, nitrofurantoin, penicillamine, procarbazine, bleomyin, vinblastine, propylthiouracil, and sulfonamides.[2,4,34] Common drugs that have been reported to cause pulmonary

Table 9-5	Drug-induced Noncardiogenic Pulmonary Edema	

Analgesic agents	Antimicrobial agents	Cardiovascular agents
Acetylsalicylic acid*	Amphotericin B	Amiodarone*
Morphine (agonists/ antagonists)*	Cotrimoxazole	Acetazolamide
	Erythromycin	Adrenaline
Sulfasalazine*	Minocycline*	Diltiazem
Codeine	Pyrimethamine-sulfadoxine	Hydrochlorothiazide
Colchicine	Sulfamides-sulfonamides*	Nicardipine
Ibuprofen		Nitroglycerin
Methadone	**Obs–Gyne agents**	Nitric oxide
Oxycodone	Beta-agonists (IV in Obs/ Gyne)*	Propranolol
Para-(4)-aminosalicylic acid	Clomiphene	Prostacyclin
Chemotherapeutic/ immunosuppressant agents	Medroxyprogesterone	Phenylephrine
Anti-lymphocyte (thymocyte) globulin	Salbutamol*	**Miscellanous agents**
	Tamoxifen	Heroin*
Basiliximab	Terbutaline	Iodine, radiographic contrast media*
Cyclosporin	**Neurological agents**	Propofol
Cytokines	Carbamazepine*	Protamine
Cytarabine arabinoside	Ergometrine	Quinine
Cyclophosphamide*	Ritodrine	
Dexamethasone	**Endocrine agents**	
Doxorubicin	Deferoxamine	
Gemcitabine	Insulin	
Interleukin 2	Lipids	
Immunoglobulins (IV)	Ornipressin	
Methotrexate*	Metamizole	
Immune globulin	Pioglitazone	
Propoxyphene/ dextropropoxyphene	Rosiglitazone	
Rituximab	Thiazolidinediones	
Paclitaxel	Troglitazone	
TNF-alfa	Vasopressin	
Vinorelbine		

*Denotes drugs most commonly cited for a toxicity pattern of noncardiogenic pulmonary edema.

edema without diffuse alveolar damage include NSAIDs, salicylates, and colony-stimulating factors.[35] Clinical and radiographic manifestations are indistinguishable from other causes of ARDS and pulmonary edema.[36,37]

The typical clinical presentation of noncardiogenic pulmonary edema is the acute onset of hypoxia, dyspnea, and tachypnea. Chest radiographs, in the setting

Table 9-6	Drug-induced ARDS
Common	**Rare**
Amiodarone	Acetylsalicylic acid
Cyclophosphamide	Aminoglutethimide
BCG therapy	Bleomycin
Gefitinib	Bortezomib
Gemcitabine	Carbamazepine
Rituximab	Cetuximab
Transfusion of plasma containing blood products	Cytarabine (cytosine arabinoside)
	Etoposide
	Everolimus
	Interferon gamma
	Mercaptopurine
	Methotrexate
	Morphine (agonists/antagonists)
	Nitrofurantoin
	Nitrosoureas
	Oxaliplatin
	Pranlukast
	Radiation
	Simvastatin
	Sirolimus
	Ticlopidine
	Topotecan

of pulmonary edema without diffuse alveolar damage, are similar to hydrostatic pulmonary edema; however, unlike pulmonary edema, due to congestive heart failure, cardiomegaly, and pulmonary vascular blood flow redistribution is often absent in the setting of drug-induced causes. In diffuse alveolar damage, ground-glass opacities and areas of consolidation are seen in the posterior and dependent regions of the lung.[36,37] On histologic examination, the presence of hyaline membranes is characteristic of the exudative stage of ARDS. After seven days, the organized or fibroproliferative stage of ARDS ensues. There is reabsorption of hyaline membranes; and overall, the histology is consistent with organizing pneumonia.

For most of the agents, the pathogenic mechanisms responsible for ARDS and pulmonary edema are unknown and idiosyncratic. Most agents responsible for this type of toxicity are unrelated to drug dosages and duration of therapy. Accepted pathogenic mechanisms include drug-induced capillary leak, anaphylaxis, and hypervolemia.

A lung biopsy is rarely performed, but when it is obtained, it is often nonspecific. Diagnostic tests of exclusion of other disorders that have a similar presentation such as congestive heart failure, pulmonary hemorrhage, or infection are performed.

Although fatal drug reactions are reported, most cases of drug-induced pulmonary edema/ARDS are self-limited and recovery is typically rapid with drug discontinuation. Mechanical ventilation may be needed. Diuretic therapy has been used in the setting of noncardiogenic pulmonary edema; however, it should be used under caution, as it may adversely affect outcomes. Systemic corticosteroids have been used with reported success; however, their therapeutic role remains unknown.

Diffuse Alveolar Hemorrhage and Vasculitis

Several drugs have been implicated in the development of diffuse alveolar hemorrhage (DAH) with or without capillaritis. Bland hemorrhage without vasculitis often occurs in the setting of anticoagulant therapy, but it also has been described with amiodarone and cyclophosphamide. Systemic small vessel vasculitis has been described mostly with propylthiouracil; a positive p-ANCA is typically present. Rare reports of p-ANCA-associated small vessel vasculitis have been described with sulfasalazine, retinoic acid, interferon, methimazole, simvastatin, anti-TNF therapy, and diphenylhydantoin. Ground-glass opacities with areas of consolidation may be scattered and diffused on chest imaging. Ill-defined centrilobular nodules and crazy-paving pattern (intralobar and interlobular septal thickening with superimposed ground-glass opacities) may be seen on HRCT.

The clinical presentation of drug-induced DAH is usually acute and often results in respiratory failure requiring mechanical ventilation. It is characterized by the accumulation of red blood cells in the alveolar spaces. The origin of the red blood cells is thought to be from alveolar capillaries and less frequently from precapillary arterioles or postcapillary venules.[38] Patients have varying degrees of hemoptysis, cough, and dyspnea. However, the cardinal symptom of hemoptysis is absent in one-third of cases.[39] A decreasing hemoglobin level on laboratory evaluation and a progressive, hemorrhagic, bronchoalveolar lavage is noted in sequential samples. The mechanisms for drug-induced DAH may involve an immune/hypersensitivity reaction, direct cytotoxic effect on the alveolar capillary basement membrane, or a coagulation defect.

Several distinct histopathologies have been described with drug-induced DAH. Pulmonary capillaritis has been described with all-trans-retinoic acid, propylthiouracil, and diphenylhydantoin.[39,40-42] In addition, penicillamine, hydralazine, and carbimazole can induce a systemic vasculitis picture with DAH and glomerulonephritis.[43-48] This histology can also be seen in Wegener's granulomatosis, microscopic polyangitis, cryoglobulinemia, and other connective tissue disorders such as systemic lupus erythematosus. An autoimmune or hypersensitivity reaction is believed to be the mechanism for drug-induced pulmonary capillaritis.

Another pulmonary hypersensitivity reaction is HUS, which may be induced by mitomycin treatment.[49] HUS occurs in 2–10% of patients treated with mitomycin. The clinical presentation of mitomycin-induced HUS consists of microangiopathic hemolytic anemia with fragmentation of the red blood cells, renal failure, neurological problems, fever, and diffuse pulmonary infiltrates. Blood transfusions should be avoided as they may potentate the syndrome (Table 9-7).

Pulmonary veno-occlusive disease (PVOD) with accompanying DAH has been reported as a complication of chemotherapy. Bleomycin and carmustine appear to be the most common cause of drug-induced PVOD. Mitomycin-C, gemcitabine, and vinca alkaloids have also been implicated.[49-51]

Table 9-7 Drug-induced Diffuse Alveolar Hemorrhage	
Common	**Rare**
Acetylsalicylic acid	Sulfasalazine*
Amiodarone	Busulfan*
Anticoagulants	Simvastatin***
Carbamazepine	Hydralazine***
Methotrexate	Methimazole***
Mitomycin-C	Interferon***
Propylthiouracil	Atorvastatin***
Nitrofurantoin	Minocycline***
Sirolimus/tacrolimus	Anti-TNF alfa agents***
Penicillamine**	Cephotaxime***
	Diphenylhydantoin***
	Pantoprazole***
	All-trans-retinoic acid***
	Fibrinolytics
	Cytarabine
	Clopidrogel
	Azathioprine
	Alemtuzumab*
	Infliximab***
	Moxalactam
	Quinidine
	Rituximab
	Valproic acid
	Carbimazole**

*Denotes drugs associated with a Goodpasture's reaction only.
**Denotes drugs associated with both a Goodpasture's reaction and p-ANCA vasculitis.
***Denotes drugs associated with a p-ANCA vasculitis only.

Direct lung epithelial cell toxicity, leading to ARDS, has been attributed to several drugs. During the exudative phase of drug-induced ARDS, DAH may occur. Amiodarone, nitrofurantoin, and freebasing cocaine can result in DAH by direct lung injury.[38,52-54]

Finally, a bland pulmonary hemorrhage in which the lung interstitium is not inflamed and the pulmonary vessels are normal may occur in drug-induced DAH. Drugs that interfere with platelet function or coagulation, or cause drug-induced thrombocytopenia are typical causes in this setting, especially if coexisting pulmonary venous hypertension or pneumonia is present.[55-61]

Eosinophilic Pneumonia

Several diseases exist in which the lung contains an abnormal concentration of eosinophils. Clinically encountered eosinophilic lung diseases include simple pulmonary eosinophilia; acute eosinophilic pneumonia; chronic eosinophilic pneumonia; Churg-Strauss syndrome; asthma; allergic bronchopulmonary mycosis; parasite-induced pulmonary eosinophilia; hypereosinophilic syndrome; fungal-induced pulmonary eosinophilia; and drug-induced pulmonary eosinophilia.[62,63] It is important to exclude these diseases during the initial clinical evaluation of suspected eosinophilic lung diseases.

Drug toxicity is an important cause of acute and chronic eosinophilic pneumonia. Serum eosinophilia most often accompanies cases of chronic eosinophilic pneumonia. In acute eosinophilic pneumonia, the clinical and radiographic presentation is often similar to ARDS with the development of fulminant hypoxic respiratory failure. In contrast, the clinical presentation of chronic eosinophilic pneumonia is subacute to chronic. The distribution of the parenchymal infiltrates is peripherally distributed in the chronic form. In drug-induced cases of eosinophilic pneumonia, patterns of acute lung injury, overlapping diffuse alveolar damage, are typically noted.

Commonly reported drug-induced pulmonary eosinophilia has been noted with amiodarone, bleomycin, captopril, gold salts, radiocontrast agents, L-tryptophan, methotrexate, nitrofurantoin, and phenytoin.[64-69] Drugs that are occasionally reported to cause pulmonary eosinophilia include acetylsalicylic acid, carbamazepine, GM-CSF, minocycline, nilutamide, penicillamine, propylthiouracil, sulfa-containing medications, and sulfasalazine. Rare reports of drug-induced eosinophilia include NSAIDs, acetaminophen, enalapril, hydralazine, penicillin, ranitidine, zafirlukast, imipramine, ampicillin, phenylbutazone, procarbazine, streptomycin, tetracycline, and trazodone.[2,70-76] In perspective of the clinical and radiographic presentation, eosinophilic pneumonia is diagnosed by demonstrating greater than 25% eosinophils on BAL.

Churg-Strauss syndrome (CSS) presents with asthma, serum eosinophilia, and granulomatosis vasculitis. CSS has been linked to leukotriene inhibitors, including montelukast and zifirlukast.[77-79] In drug-related CSS, antecedent asthma and allergic rhinitis were present with a presentation of high blood eosinophilia and vasculitis, involving the peripheral nerves, skin, heart, lung, kidney, and gastrointestinal tract. It is unclear if leukotriene inhibitors cause CSS. Some have speculated that leukotriene inhibitors were used as steroid-sparing agents, allowing for the development of occult CSS to clinically manifest when steroids were tapered.[77-79]

Granulomatosis Pneumonitis

Granulomatous inflammation of the lung can develop from infectious (mycobacterial or fungal infections) or from noninfectious causes including sarcoidosis, hypersensitivity pneumonitis, and drugs. When necrosis is noted, infectious causes should be strongly considered. Drug-induced granulomatosis pneumonitis has been associated with TNF alfa therapy; acebutol; cocaine; cromolyn sodium; fluoxetine; methotrexate; nitrofurantoin; procarbazine; pentazocine; sirolimus; and intravesical Bacillus Calmette Guerin (BCG) therapy for the treatment of bladder cancer.[2,9] Anti-TNF alfa treatment is the most likely cause of granulomatosis pneumonitis (Table 9-8). Bronchiolitis and interstitial inflammation, similar to hypersensitivity pneumonitis, have been described in drug-related scenarios. It remains problematic in BCG-related granulomatosis pneumonitis whether the granulomas form as a result of systemic dissemination of the mycobacteria or as a result of an over-exuberant immune response.[80]

Infliximab, etanercept, and adalimumab are the three commercially available anti-TNF alfa medications approved in the United States. The drugs are commonly used in the treatment of Cohn's disease, psoriasis, rheumatoid arthritis, and ankylosing spondylitis. The most common adverse event associated with these drugs is related to their immunomodulating effects, predisposing the patient to increased infections including opportunistic pathogens and tuberculosis. The most common DILI associated with these agents is interstitial pneumonitis and pulmonary fibrosis (reported rates of 0.5–0.6% of at-risk patients). Interestingly, a sarcoid-like reaction with anti-TNF alfa therapy has been reported with all three commercially available drugs. The frequency of this reaction is reported in 0.04% of treated cases with a

Table 9-8	Drug-induced Granulomatosis Pneumonitis	
Anti-TNF alfa therapy*	Methotrexate
BCG	Sirolimus
Etanercept	Leflunomide
Interferon	

*Denotes drug most commonly cited for drug-induced granulomatosis pneumonitis.

median time of clinical presentation of 18 months. The most frequent radiographic presentation is pulmonary opacities with hilar and mediastinal lymphadenopathy. Noncaseating granulomas have been documented on fine-needle aspiration of mediastinal lymph nodes, transbronchial biopsy of lung tissue as well as skin biopsy. Improvement was observed in all cases with drug discontinuation with or without corticosteroids. Some reports have described that alternate anti-TNF agents did not result in relapse of the condition.[81-87]

Cough and Bronchospasm

Cough is a frequent symptom of drug-induced lung disease and can occur as a lone mechanism in DILI. The most common medication implicated in the development of an isolated cough is angiotensin converting enzyme inhibitors (ACEI). ACEI can cause an isolated dry cough in the absence of bronchospasm. ACEI-related cough has been reported to occur in 5–35% of patients using the medication.[88] The cough can develop anytime during the use of ACEI and is not dose-related. ACEI-induced inhibition of bradykinin metabolism is considered to be the mechanism by which ACEI-induced cough occurs.[89] While the cough typically resolves 1–4 weeks after discontinuing the medication, complete resolution may not occur for three months.[90] Angiotensin-II antagonists are a good alternative and rarely induce cough. Cough has also been reported with fentanyl and methotrexate.[91-93]

Drug toxicity may affect both large and small airways. Drug-induced broncho-constriction is caused by various agents and is reversible (Table 9-9). Patients typically have cough, wheezing, and dyspnea soon after exposure to the agent. Aspirin, NSAIDs, and beta-blockers are common causative agents. This is especially

Table 9-9	Drug-induced Cough and Bronchospasm	
Lone cough	**Bronchospasm**	
	Common	*Rare*
ACEIs	Salicylates	Propofol
Methotrexate	ACEIs	Oxaliplatin
Fentanyl	NSAIDs	Paclitaxel
Morphine	Amiodarone	Penicillin
	Beta-blockers	Vinblastine
	Carbamazepine	
	Nitrofurantoin	
	Salbutamol	
	Pentamidine	
	Contrast media	
	Sulfonamides	

ACEI, angiotensin converting enzyme inhibitors.

true for asthmatics who have allergies to NSAIDs or aspirin. Rarely, bronchospasm can occur after the use of adenosine.[94] Drug-induced bronchospasm is typically reversible after the use of bronchodilators, but in some cases, it can be severe. In a single report, drug-induced bronchospasm accounted for 14% of severe sudden bronchospasm in the intensive care unit (ICU) settings.[95] Patients without a history of underlying asthma may develop this reaction. Inhaled pentamidine causes bronchospasm in 24–40% of patients.[96] Symptoms of bronchospasm can be prevented with preadministration of a bronchodilator.

Drug-induced Pleural Disease

Drug-induced pleural disease is an uncommon occurrence in contrast to drug-induced parenchymal lung disease.[97-99] However, as new drugs are developed, an increasing number of drugs implicated in the development of pleural disease should be anticipated. These drugs may incite a pleural reaction alone or in conjunction with parenchymal disease. The presentation of drug-induced pleural disease varies from an asymptomatic pleural effusion, acute pleuritis, symptomatic pleural thickening, and systemic presentations with DIL. Except in some cases of DIL pleuritis, the pathogenic mechanism for most of the drug-induced pleural disease remains speculative. These mechanisms include a hypersensitivity or allergic reaction; a direct toxic effect; increased oxygen free radical production; suppression of antioxidant defenses; and chemical-induced inflammation.[97]

Approximately 70 drugs are believed to cause pleural diseases.[2] These includes cardiovascular agents such as practolol, amiodarone, and minoxidil; ergoline drugs such as methysergide and bromocriptine; sclerotherapy agents such as sodium morrhuate and alcohol; and chemotherapeutic agents such as docetaxel, bleomycin, mitomycin, procarbazine, methotrexate, cyclophosphamide, and tyrosine kinase inhibitors (Table 9-10). Other classes of drugs have been associated with pleural effusions and a laundry list of drugs implicated in DIL pleuritis has been reported (Table 9-11). Pleural thickening with or without pleural effusion may be a manifestation of drug toxicity.

In the majority of cases related to drug-induced pleural effusion, a pleural fluid analysis shows a lymphocyte predominant, concordant exudate. Recently, we described two cases of chylous effusions occurring as a complication of dasatinib.[100] Pleural fluid analysis was consistent with a protein-discordant exudate with lymphocyte predominance. The presence of chylomicrons consistent with a chyle leak was noted in both the cases. This was the first case series describing a drug-induced syndrome similar to the clinical presentation of yellow nail syndrome.[100]

Pleural fluid eosinophilia (defined as > 10% of the nucleated cells) should suggest the possibility of drug-induced pleural disease; however, its presence or absence is a nonspecific finding. The important causes of pleural fluid eosinophilia include

Table 9-10	Drug-induced Pleural Effusions	
Antimicrobial agents		**Endocrine agents**
Acyclovir		Clomiphene
Dapsone		Rosiglitazone
Navirapine		Troglitazone
Nitrofurantoin		Propylthiouracil
Penicillamine		
Praziquantel		**Tyrosine kinase inhibitors***
Sulfamides-sulfonamides		Dasatinib
		Gefitinib
Cardiovascular agents		Imatinib
Acebutolol		
Amiodarone		**Neurological/psychiatric agents**
Carvedilol		Bromocriptine
Hydralazine		Cabergoline
Pravastatin		Clozapine
Propranolol		Dihydroergocristine
Minoxidil		Dihydroergotamine
Simvastatin		Ergotamine
Procainamide		Ethchlorvynol
		Lisuride
Chemotherapeutic agents		Methysergide
Carmustine (BCNU)		Nicergoline
Cyclophosphamide		Pergolide
Daunorubicin		Phenytoin
Docetaxel		
Methotrexate		
Procarbazine		

*Pleural effusions occurring in the setting of tyrosine kinase therapy are typically protein discordant exudates. Chylous effusions have also been described.

pneumothorax, hemothorax, benign asbestos pleural effusion, fungal disease, Hodgkin's lymphoma, pulmonary emboli with pulmonary infarction, and parasitic infection.[97] These diseases are important to exclude prior to consider the diagnosis of drug-induced pleural disease. More than 20 drugs have been documented to cause pleural fluid eosinophilia[2] (Table 9-12). Systemic eosinophilia may not always be present.

Since the initial description of a lupus-like illness following treatment with sulfadiazine in 1945 by Hoffman,[101] more than 80 drugs are reported to cause a lupus-like reaction or exacerbate pre-existing lupus.[2] However, only a small number of drugs have a strong association with DIL, they include procainamide, hydralazine, chlorpromazine, isoniazid, D-pencillamine, methyldopa, and quinidine.[101-103]

Table 9-11	Drug-induced Lupus	
Strongly associated with lupus pleuritis	**Cardiovascular agents**	**Gynecological agents**
Chlorpromazine	Acebutolol	Danazol
Hydralazine	Amiodarone, atenolol	Oral contraceptives
Isoniazid	Captopril	**Immune modulators**
Methyldopa	Clonidine	Gold salts
Penicillamine	Disopyramide	Interferon (alfa, gamma)
Procainamide	Labetalol	**Neurological agents**
Quinidine	Lovastatin	Levo-dopa
Anticonvulsants	Minoxidil	Methylsergide
Carbamazepine	Practolol	**Oncologic agent**
Ethosuximide	Prinolol	Leuprolide acetate
Primidone	Spironolactone	**Ophthalmological agent**
Anti-inflammatory agents	**Endocrine agents**	Timolol eyedrops
Diclofenac	Aminoglutethimide	**Psychiatric agent**
Ibuprofen	Methimazole	Lithium carbonate
Para-aminosalicylic acid	Propylthiouracil	
Sulindac	**Gastrointestinal agents**	
Tolmetin	Promethazine	
	Sulfasalazine	

Table 9-12	Drug-induced Pleural Fluid Eosinophilia
Acebutolol	Imidapril
Acyclovir	Infliximab
Antidepressants*	Isotretinoin*
Beta-blockers*	Mesalamine*
Clozapine	Practolol*
Dantrolene	Propylthiouracil*
Diltiazem	Simvastatin*
Divalproex sodium	Sulfasalazine*
Fenfluramine/dexfenfluramine*	Tizanidine
Fluoxetine	Trimipramine*
Gliclazide	Valproic acid

*Denotes drugs most commonly implicated in the development of a drug-induced pleural fluid eosinophilia.

Pleuropulmonary involvement is especially common in DIL. Approximately 56% of patients with procainamide-induced lupus have pleural effusions and pleuritis.[101] In approximately 30% of patients with hydralazine-induced lupus, pleuropulmonary disease is reported.[101] The pleural fluid characteristics of DIL which are similar to idiopathic lupus include effusions which are exudative with cell counts of 200–15,000 cells/µl; pleural fluid pH and glucose are usually normal but may be low in less than 15% of cases; pleural fluid antinuclear antibodies (ANA) are higher than concomitant serum values and titers frequently exceed 1:250; and a cytological examination may reveal the diagnostic presence of LE cells.[102] Antihistone antibodies are not specific for DIL and can be found in 50–80% of patients with native lupus. Antihistone antibodies can be detected in rheumatoid arthritis, Felty's syndrome, and mixed connective tissue diseases.[101-103]

Hypocomplementemia and anti-double stranded DNA are seen in less than 1% of DIL in comparison to native lupus where the frequency is 66% and 44%, respectively.[101] Intrinsic renal disease is extremely rare in DIL as compared to idiopathic lupus.

In conclusion, drug-induced pleural disease is relatively uncommon and less appreciated by clinicians than drug-induced parenchymal lung disease. Pleural reactions from drugs manifest as pleural effusions, pleural thickening, or pleuritic chest pain, and may occur in the absence of parenchymal infiltrates. The clinician should be cognizant of the possibility of a drug-induced pleural reaction. A detailed drug history, temporal relationship between symptom onset and initiation of therapy, and pleural fluid eosinophilia should raise the suspicion of a drug-related process. If the cause of an exudative pleural effusion is not clinically obvious, drug therapy withdrawal should be considered prior to initiate an extensive diagnostic evaluation.

DIAGNOSIS AND TREATMENT

It is imperative for the clinician to maintain a high index of suspicion to make an accurate diagnosis of DILI. The differential diagnosis is broad; however, it can be narrowed by recognition of specific clinical and radiographic patterns. An extensive review of the medication history including prescribed over the counter medications, illicit drugs, radiation exposure, and herbal-vitamin supplements must be performed. Drug exposure must precede onset of clinical symptoms. The time to develop DILI may be within a few minutes such as drug-induced bronchospasm following aspirin exposure; however, it may not develop for several years as with chemotherapy or nitrofurantoin-induced pulmonary fibrosis.

Symptoms vary from cough and insidious dyspnea to fulminant presentations of acute hypoxic respiratory failure. In most cases of DILI, toxicity is limited to the lungs; however, extrapulmonary symptoms may occur with drug-induced lupus or drug-induced vasculitis. Diagnostic criteria for DILI include: a history of drug exposure; clinical, imaging, and histopathological pattern consistent with prior observations of drug reactions; exclusion of other potential etiologies such as pulmonary infection, cardiogenic and noncardiogenic pulmonary edema, and pulmonary involvement due to systemic disease and malignancy; improvement following discontinuation of the suspected drug; and recurrence of symptoms upon rechallenge to elicit the same toxicity pattern remains the gold standard to establish DILI. Unfortunately, a rechallenge test may not be possible to give the severity of the clinical presentation; with methotrexate-induced pneumonitis, rechallenge may decrease the likelihood of toxicity.[3]

The standard testing for evaluation of DILI includes chest radiograph, pulmonary function tests (PFTs), and HRCT. In most of the cases, invasive testing with bronchoscopy and bronchoalveolar lavage (BAL) with or without transbronchial biopsies is performed. In limited and highly selective cases, a surgical lung biopsy may be performed. PFTs may show an obstructive ventilatory defect with acute bronchospasm or bronchiolitis obliterans. A restrictive defect, suggestive on spirometry or confirmed with lung volumes with decreased diffusing capacity for carbon monoxide, is seen in cases of interstitial pneumonitis and pulmonary fibrosis. With alveolar hemorrhage, the diffusing capacity is increased due to the presence of intra-alveolar red blood cells. HRCT better defines the pattern and distribution of parenchymal involvement as compared to the chest radiography and helps to narrow the differential diagnosis. Other noninvasive studies, which may be considered, include an echocardiogram, sputum Gram's stain and culture, and serologic testing in cases of suspected vasculitis and connective tissue diseases.[3]

In most of the cases with parenchymal involvement, pulmonologists will perform bronchoscopy with BAL to exclude an alternative diagnosis. BAL has a high diagnostic yield for pulmonary infection and may exclude malignancy, especially when combined with biopsies.[104] Therefore, BAL is useful in eliminating alternative diagnoses as the cause of lung disease, if the BAL results are consistent with the clinician suspicion. Findings may, however, support the diagnosis of DILI. The cellular pattern of BAL may be nonspecific; however, the differential diagnosis can be narrowed with specific diagnosis as noted in table 9-13.

Table 9-13	Bronchoalveolar Lavage Findings in Drug-induced Lung Injury
Drug-induced lung disease	*Findings*
Cytotoxic reactions; diffuse alveolar damage	Atypcial and hyperplastic type II pneumocytes; BAL neutrophilia
Diffuse alveolar hemorrhage	Hemosiderin-laden macrophages; progressively bloody lavage returns red blood cell fragments in macrophages
Hypersensitivity pneumonitis	BAL lymphocytosis; CD4/CD8 < 1
Eosinophilic pneumonia	Eosinophils > 25%
Alveolar proteinosis	Milky effluent; Periodic Acid-Schiff positive corpuscles; foamy macrophages

The cellular pattern of the BAL can be lymphocytic, neutrophilic, eosinophilic, or mixed celluarity. Understanding the celluarity of the BAL fluid is helpful in limiting the differential diagnosis. In disease processes that create a lymphocytosis, the differential diagnosis can be further narrowed by examining the CD4/CD8 ratio.[105] An increased CD4/CD8 ratio in the setting of a lymphocytic alveolitis is seen with sarcoidosis, berylliosis, alveolar proteinosis, Crohn's disease, and connective-tissue disorders. A normal CD4/CD8 ratio is seen with tuberculosis and malignant infiltrates with or without lymphangitic carcinomatosis. A decreased CD4/CD8 ratio has been observed with drug-induced pneumonitis, cryptogenic organizing pneumonia (COP)—a hypersensitivity reaction, silicosis, and HIV infection.[105] Table 9-14 describes the cellular pattern on BAL with the differential diagnoses.

Table 9-14	Bronchoalveolar Lavage Cellular Pattern with Drug-induced Lung Injury
Cellular pattern	*Diagnosis*
Lymphocytosis	Hypersensitivity pneumonitis
	Drug-induced pneumonitis
	Sarcoidosis
	Berylliosis
	Connective-tissue disorders
	Malignant infiltrates
	Crohn's disease
	Viral pneumonia
	Silicosis
	HIV infection
	Tuberculosis
	Primary biliary cirrhosis
Neutrophilia	Acute respiratory distress syndrome
	Acute interstitial pneumonia
	Idiopathic pulmonary fibrosis
	Desquamative interstitial pneumonia
	Bacterial pneumonia
	Bronchiolitis obliterans
	Diffuse panbronchiolitis
	Wegener's granulomatosis
	Connective-tissue disorders
	Asbestosis
	Drug-induced pneumonitis

Continued

Continued

Cellular pattern	Diagnosis
Eosinophilia	Eosinophilic pneumonia
	Churg-Strauss syndrome
	Hypereosinophilic syndrome
	Drug-induced pneumonitis
	Allergic bronchopulmonary mycosis
Mixed cellularity	Bronchiolitis obliterans with organizing pneumonia
	Nonspecific interstitial pneumonia
	Inorganic dust exposure
	Drug-induced pneumonitis
	Connective-tissue disorders

In drug-induced hypersensitivity pneumonitis, the typical BAL findings include lymphocytosis > 50%; a CD4/CD8 ratio < 1; and at times, an increase in neutrophils. Eosinophilic pneumonia classically has an elevated eosinophil count in the BAL fluid of > 25%.[62,63] BAL findings with cytotoxic pneumonitis show a neutrophil predominance. BAL findings in drug-induced organizing pneumonia are relatively nonspecific; however, the total nucleated cell count usually shows mixed celluarity. BAL findings in drug-induced DAH reveal hemosiderin-laden macrophages as well as increasingly bloody return from repetitive lavages.[105] On cytologic examination, the presence of foamy macrophages and gold in the cytoplasm of macrophages only indicate drug exposure to amiodarone and gold salts, respectively; they do not necessarily establish drug toxicity.[98] Transbronchial lung biopsy may support a diagnosis of drug-induced parenchymal insult; however, these findings are often nonspecific. Surgical lung biopsy provides a higher diagnostic yield.[105] In a study reported by Cockerill and colleagues, 20% of patients with diffuse infiltrates who underwent surgical lung biopsy had pathologic findings that could be attributed to drug reaction.[104]

When DILI is suspected and all competing diagnoses have been excluded, the suspected medication should be discontinued. In the majority of cases of DILI, symptoms remit with drug removal and supportive care. With drug-induced organizing pneumonia, eosinophilic pneumonia and hypersensitivity pneumonitis, systemic corticosteroids, and steroid-sparing immunosuppressive agents hasten resolution of symptoms. In contrast, systemic corticosteroids do not appear to have any therapeutic role in drug-induced pulmonary fibrosis, pulmonary vascular disease, and bronchiolitis obliterans, and disease progression may continue despite drug removal.[3]

CASE STUDY 1

A 51-year-old man having a mixed connective tissue disease with associated intestinal lung disease presented with a three-day history of dyspnea, fever, and cough. His most recent pulmonary function tests demonstrated a severe restrictive defect, and the diffusing capacity for carbon monoxide was significantly reduced. He demonstrated clinical progression of his interstitial lung disease despite pulse dose cyclophosphamide for six months and was started on rituximab. His medications at presentation included prednisone 15 mg daily, azathioprine 100 mg daily, and he was given a dose of rituximab three weeks prior.

On presentation, his temperature was 101.6 °F, pulse rate 110/minute, respiratory rate 36/minute, blood pressure 145/85 mmHg, and oxygen saturation of 75% on room air. Physical examination was noted for diffuse, non-velcro crackles. Otherwise, his physical examination was noncontributory. He was emergently intubated and transferred to the medical ICU for ongoing treatment.

Portable chest radiograph at presentation is shown in figure 9-1. He was started on broad-spectrum intravenous antibiotics. Bronchoscopy was performed. Bronchoalveolar lavage showed 7,800 red blood cells/µL and 1,200 total nucleated cells/µL. The differential nucleated cell count showed 70% neutrophils, 20% lymphocytes, and 10% macrophages. Cytological examination and all

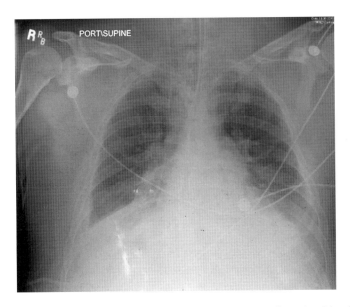

Figure 9-1 A portable chest radiograph, 30 minutes following endotracheal intubation. The endotracheal tube and a right internal jugular central line are well positioned. Diffuse bilateral alveolar opacities are present. Small bilateral pleural effusions are also noted.

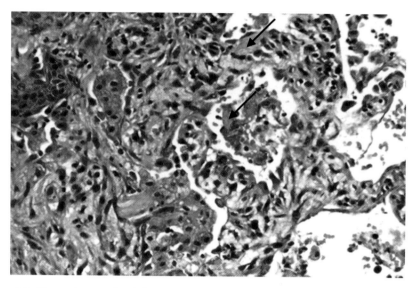

Figure 9-2 Photomicrograph of the VATS-surgical lung biopsy is shown. Findings are consistent with ARDS in the exudative stage. Note the hyaline membrane formation (arrows) in the alveolar spaces. This is the hallmark finding for diffuse alveolar damage in the exudative stage of ARDS.

microbiologic studies, including AFB, fungal, aerobic cultures, and respiratory viral PCR, were negative. Video-assisted thoracoscopic lung biopsy was obtained. Figure 9-2 shows the hematoxylin and eosin stain of the lung biopsy specimen. He was treated with high-dose corticosteroids and was subsequently weaned from the mechanical ventilator in five days.

A clinical diagnosis of rituximab-induced ARDS was established.

CASE STUDY 2

A 68-year-old white female, nonsmoker with a history of CML presented to a pulmonary clinic upon referral from her oncologist with a two-year history of bilateral pleural effusions and a chief complaint of increasing dyspnea and a persistent cough. Ten months prior, she was started on dasatinib at 140 mg/day after failing other conventional therapies. Her past medical history was notable for chronic renal insufficiency (baseline creatinine 1.4 mg/dL), herpes-zoster, hypertension, hypothyroidism, hyperlipidemia, and an autologous stem cell transplant nine years prior. Her surgical history was noted for a remotely placed Port-a-Cath. Her medications included hydroxyurea, dasatinib 100 mg/day, synthroid 25 mcg/day, omacor twice/daily, nexium 40 mg/day, lopressor 50 mg twice/daily, folic acid 1 mg/day, and ativan 1 mg as needed.

On physical examination, the patient's vital signs were as follows: temperature 97.6 °F, pulse rate 91/minute, respiratory rate 20/minute, blood pressure 147/75 mmHg, and room air oxygen saturation at rest 97%. Cardiovascular examination demonstrated no jugular venous distension with a regular rate and rhythm without murmurs or gallops. Lung examination revealed no adventitious breath sounds. There was evidence of decreased bilateral expansion, left greater than right, and there was dullness to percussion with decreased fremitus and absent breath sounds in the bases. The abdomen was obese and nontender without hepatosplenomegaly. The extremities showed no cyanosis, clubbing, or edema.

Chest radiograph showed bilateral pleural effusions (left greater than right) with a normal cardiomediastinal silhouette without evidence of parenchymal, interstitial or alveolar infiltrates with a right indwelling central venous catheter. Bilateral thoracocenteses were performed. The pleural fluid analysis is reported in table 9-15. A diagnosis of dasatinib-induced chylous pleural effusions was established. A reduction in the dasatinib dose to 50 mg/d resulted in a reduction of the bilateral effusions and dyspnea.

Table 9-15	Pleural Fluid Analysis	
Characteristics	*Right pleural fluid analysis*	*Left pleural fluid analysis*
Appearance	Hemorrhagic/chylous	Hemorrhagic
Total nucleated cells/μL	2,007	2,683
Differential cell count (%)	91 lymphocytes, 8 macrophages, 1 mesothelial cell	96 lymphocytes, 4 macrophages
Red blood cell/μL	28,303	66,264
Total protein (g/dL)	4.4	4.6
Pleural fluid/serum protein ratio	0.60	0.68
LDH (IU/L)	109	139
pH	7.41	7.37
Amylase (IU/L)	34	35
Triglycerides (mg/dL)	155	171
Chylomicrons	Present	Present
Glucose (mg/dL)	98	94
Flow cytometry	Negative	Negative
Manometry	Normal	Normal
Cytology	Negative	Negative
Serum albumin (g/dL)	3.6	3.4
Cultures (fungus/AFB/ bacteria)	Negative	Negative

Commonly Encountered Medications

Amiodarone

Amiodarone (Am) is a bi-iodinated benzofuran derivative and is one of the most commonly prescribed medications for the treatment of ventricular and supra-ventricular arrhythmias, worldwide. Am and its metabolite, desethylamiodarone (DEAm), are cationic amphiphilics that accumulate in lung, liver, spleen, skin, thyroid, and eye. Both Am and DEAm are toxic to lung tissue, even with therapeutic serum levels. Am and DEAm localize to cell lysosomes and block the turnover of endogenous phospholipids, which account for the presence of foamy lipid-laden macrophages observed on bronchoalveolar lavage or lung biopsy specimens from patients who have taken Am for an extended period of time.

Lung toxicity associated with Am can occur as early as two days or after several years. Pulmonary toxicity of Am generally falls into two categories: lipoid pneumonia or Am effect, which is usually asymptomatic; and Am toxicity, which includes several distinct clinical entities related to various patterns of lung inflammation. Examples include ARDS, DAH, eosinophilic pneumonia, acute fibrinous organizing pneumonia (AFOP), acute DIP, chronic organizing pneumonia, a pattern similar to nonspecific interstitial pneumonia, a pattern similar to usual interstitial pneumonia and pulmonary nodules/masses.[106-116]

The incidence of subacute/chronic Am pulmonary toxicity (APT) varies subs-tantially because of different study designs and criteria used to define Am toxicity. The prevalence of Am toxicity is 5–15% in those taking 500 mg or more per day and 0.1–0.5% in those taking more than 200 mg/day. The incidence of acute APT is unkown.[99,110]

Age is one of the most important risk factors in the development of APT. APT increases to three-fold every 10 years in patients who are greater than 60 years of age as compared to those less than 60 years of age.

APT is associated with duration and intensity of exposure. The cumulative incidence of APT is 4%, 8%, and 11% at 1, 3, and 5 years of use, respectively.[106] Acute APT has been described occurring as early as the second day of exposure and for a cumulative dose as low as 1,000 mg intravenously.

Other independent risk factors in the development of chronic APT are high serum levels of DEAm, a history of cardiothoracic surgery, the use of a high FiO_2, the use of iodinated contrast media and pre-existing lung disease or the presence of coexisting pulmonary infection. In addition, abrupt withdrawal of corticosteroids has been described in the setting of acute APT.

The proposed mechanisms for APT are complex and are probably inter-connected. The mechanisms of APT include a direct cytotoxic effect of the type II pneumocytes and other intra-alveolar cells; an immune-mediated mechanism; and the activation of the angiotensin enzyme system. In an animal model of APT, an imbalance of the T helper lymphocytes subtypes (type 1 and type 2), favoring the production of transforming growth factor-beta and tumor necrosis factor-alfa have been implicated. Furthermore, *in vitro* studies have shown that Am induces alveolar cell apoptosis, which is abrogated by angiotensin II antagonists.[106]

Acute APT appears rarely in case reports, in contrast to the literature describing subacute and chronic APT. However, acute APT is largely under-recognized in those developing acute lung injuries in the postcardiac surgery setting.[110-115] Acute APT was first described in 1985 in two patients who developed fulminant respiratory failure following pulmonary angiography.[115] The histopathologic pattern of acute APT includes diffuse alveolar damage with or without alveolar bleeding, DIP, and DAH.

With the ARDS pattern, chest radiographs show patchy or diffuse infiltrates with an interstitial with or without alveolar pattern on computed tomography. The clinical presentation of acute hypoxic respiratory failure with fever, cough, dyspnea, and pleuritic chest pain often dominates. The development of an acute interstitial pneumonitis with respiratory failure has also been described with histopathological features of DAD.

Am-induced DAH has also been described in rare reports. DAH is usually related to mechanisms that are associated with the presence of antiglomerular membrane antibodies, antineutrophil cytoplasm antibodies or to immune complexes.[2]

Am has been reported as a cause of eosinophilic pneumonia. An insidious presentation, similar to chronic eosinophilic pneumonia, has been described in addition to fulminant respiratory failure mimicking acute eosinophilic pneumonia.[2]

When pulmonary toxicity is suspected, it is prudent to discontinue Am. In the setting of ARDS and those with advanced pulmonary toxicity, the addition of corticosteroids is advised, despite a lack of randomized controlled trials. The precise dose and duration of treatment have not been established; however, most regimens report 0.5–1 mg/kg of prednisone equilvalent with a gradual taper over one year. Tapering of corticosteroids depends on response of the patient and should be done cautiously because of severe relapses that have occurred with minimal reductions in corticosteroid dosage. The response time is usually seen in 1–6 months, with two months being the average time for improvement. The mortality of APT is directly related to age and severity of the presentation. Mortality in chronic APT is 10%, 20–30% in those who require hospitalization, and 50% in those with ARDS.[106]

Nitrofurantoin

Nitrofurantoin is a commonly prescribed antimicrobial drug for recurrent urinary tract infections. Pulmonary toxicity is well described and is typically acute; however, chronic pulmonary disease does occur. The most common pathological form of nitrofurantoin-related pulmonary toxicity is interstitial pneumonitis and fibrosis. The primary histological finding of nitrofurantoin-induced pneumonitis is nonspecific interstitial pneumonia; however, cases of desquamative interstitial pneumonia have been described.[117,118] Organizing pneumonia induced by nitrofurantoin is rare with seven reported cases in the literature.[119-122] Two distinct forms of nitrofurantoin-associated BOOP, fulminant and subacute, have been reported. Fulminant presentations have been associated with poor outcomes, resulting in death.[119] Mixed histologic patterns of both organizing pneumonia and desquamative interstitial pneumonia have been described in fatal cases of nitrofurantoin lung toxicity.[120]

Transfusion-related Acute Lung Injury

With a decrease in infectious transmission and bacterial contamination of transfused blood products, transfusion-related acute lung injury (TRALI) has emerged as the leading cause of transfusion-related morbidity and mortality, worldwide. Although initially described in the early 1950s, it was not until the early 1980s that the name TRALI was coined.[123-125] In this series, Popovsky and colleagues[123] demonstrated that a leuko-agglutinating antibody was causative in the development of TRALI.

In 2004, the National Heart, Lung and Blood Institute convened a working group, and a consensus definition for TRALI was created. The diagnosis of TRALI must meet the criteria for acute lung injury and included the acute onset of symptoms; a $PaO_2/FiO_2 \leq 300$ mmHg, regardless of PEEP; bilateral infiltrates on chest radiograph; and absence of congestive heart failure. In addition to meet the criteria for acute lung injury, cases of TRALI must have the onset of symptoms or signs in ≤ 6 hours after transfusion; no acute lung injury present prior to transfusion; and if alternative causes of acute lung injury exist, TRALI can be diagnosed if the clinical course of the patient suggests that acute lung injury resulted mechanistically from the transfusion. Laboratory findings were not included in the diagnostic criteria; however, transient leukopenia, leukocyte antigen-antibody mismatch between donor and recipient HLA class I and II, and increased neutrophil priming activity in the plasma of blood products have been noted with TRALI.

In the critically-ill population, 37–44% of patients receive blood products. For those who remain in the ICU for seven days or longer, up to 85% will receive blood products.[126,127] The estimated incidence of TRALI is 8% for the critically ill, who also represents the highest risk group. As acute lung injury is uncommon in the ICU, TRALI often remains an unrecognized entity. Multiple studies have shown a dose-dependent increase in acute lung injury, when controlling for other variables associated with acute lung injury as well as the severity of illness. A synergistic effect occurs when transfusions are given in conditions that predispose the patient to acute lung injury such as sepsis or aspiration. In light of these findings, some experts have advocated a more liberal definition of TRALI to encompass those who develop acute lung injury 6–72 hours after transfusion regardless of the presence of other comorbid conditions which may elicit a lung injury response.

In a prospective trial of 225 patients admitted to an ICU due to gastrointestinal bleeding, the incidence of TRALI was 17% and increased to 27% in patients with end-stage liver disease.[128] This study affirms a high incidence of TRALI in critically-ill patients and suggests that certain diseased states, such as end-stage liver disease, may have a unique predisposition for the development of TRALI. An alternative explanation for the higher incidence of TRALI in cirrhotic versus noncirrhotic-related gastrointestinal bleeding may be attributed to the higher quantity of blood products and the increased use of fresh frozen plasma in the cirrhotic group.

TRALI is more common with plasma-containing blood products. A report from the Red Cross TRALI surveillance system reported that fresh frozen plasma (FFP) was the etiological agent in 75% of cases and 63% of the TRALI-related deaths. In most of the studies, plasma containing blood products, especially FFP, predisposed the patient to a higher risk for TRALI when compared to packed red blood cells. The development of TRALI increases mortality rates. In the noncritically-ill population, TRALI-related mortality ranges from 9 to 15%; however, in the critically-ill, TRALI mortality is reported to be as high as 41%.

The pathophysiology of TRALI supports a two-event model. The first event requires the pulmonary vascular endothelium to be activated by proinflammatory cytokines allowing for neutrophil priming and adherence. The second event ensues with the transfusion of antibodies to neutrophil antigens, infusion of bioactive lipids or soluble CD40 ligand mediating neutrophil activation and degranulation. This event leads to capillary leak, endothelium damage, and acute lung injury. Another pathogenic model of TRALI theorizes that antibody-antigen complexes, are made to form on endothelial cells, which are then scavenged by the Fc receptors of neutrophils resulting in neutrophil activation and endothelial cell injury. An alternative hypothesis suggests that TRALI does not require the presence of neutrophils. This model suggests that permeability factors, such as vascular endothelial growth factor, increase permeability of the capillary membrane that results in the development of noncardiogenic pulmonary edema.[129-133]

Residual neutrophils in blood products can potentially increase the risk of TRALI; therefore, leukoreduction may reduce the risk of TRALI. Unfortunately, *in vitro* and *in vivo* data do not support a risk reduction in TRALI with leukoreduction. Several studies have shown a correlation between the age of blood products and the risk of TRALI. However, more prospective clinical trials are needed to determine the effect of storage duration on TRALI risk and outcome.

Alloantibodies to neutrophils are associated with severe TRALI. Multiparity in female donors directly correlated to the presence of alloantibodies. In a prospective study of 8,171 blood donors in the United States, a 17% incidence of HLA antibody presence was seen in female donors. The prevalence increased with the number of pregnancies. Elimination of female donors from the plasma donor pool has shown differences in the incidence of TRALI; however, better multicentered and randomized controlled trials are needed to justify this finding.[134-136]

Treatment of TRALI is mainly supportive and using appropriate lung protective strategies for those who require positive pressure ventilation. The best strategies remain prevention and applying restricted guidelines for the administration of blood products. Restricted FFP may have the largest benefit because of its inherent risk of TRALI compared to other blood products. Better studies are needed in the future to examine different FFP transfusions-strategies in the critically-ill population.

Biological Targeted Therapies

Epidermal Growth Factor Receptor Tyrosine Kinase Inhibitors

Erlotinib and gefitinib are two human epidermal growth factor receptor (EGFR) tyrosine kinase inhibitors approved for the treatment of locally advanced and metastatic non-small cell lung cancer after failure of at least one prior chemotherapy regimen. Interstitial pneumonitis occurs in approximately 1–2% of patients and usually manifests in the first three months of starting gefitinib.[137-140] Fatal and near-fatal cases of erlotinib-induced ARDS have been cited. The mortality of gefitinib-induced pneumonitis is approximately 33%. Similarly, erlotinib-related pneumonitis is rare, occurring in about 1% of cases. The clinical presentation is typically an ARDS pattern. The mechanisms surrounding EGFR-tyrosine kinase inhibitors inducing pulmonary toxicity remain unknown. In a retrospective study conducted by the West Japan Thoracic Oncology Group, several risk factors in those susceptible to gefitinib-induced pneumonitis were identified. These risk factors included male sex; smoking history; pre-existing interstitial lung disease; pulmonary infection; congestive heart failure; lymphangitic carcinomatosis; prior thoracic radiotherapy; and prior chemotherapy with gemcitabine/cisplatin, bevacizumab, and docetaxel.[139]

There is increasing evidence that the use of EGFR inhibitors induce acute lung injury with interstitial fibrosis. According to the available literature of the EGFR inhibitors, gefitinib and erlotinib have been shown to have the maximum literature to support pulmonary toxicity. However, a case of cetuximab-induced organizing pneumonia was described in a 78-year-old man who received cetuximab and irinotecan two months prior to the treatment of metastatic colorectal carcinoma.[141]

Imatinib, a potent tyrosine kinase inhibitor, is used in the treatment of chronic myelogenous leukemia and GI stromal tumors. Imatinib-related pulmonary toxicity occurs in 0.2–1.3% of patients and usually present within 10–282 days from time of drug exposure.[4,142-145] Dyspnea due to imatinib is primarily related to fluid retention and pulmonary edema. However, cases of severe pneumonitis have been described. Fever, blood eosinophilia, dyspnea, diffuse ground-glass opacities with consolidation, and fine nodular opacities have been described on radiographic studies. Resolution of imatinib-induced pneumonitis has been reported with the use of corticosteroids.[145]

Rituximab

Rituximab is a chimeric, monoclonal IgG directed against B-cell specific CD20 antigen. It is commonly used in the treatment of non-Hodgkin's lymphoma, rheumatoid arthritis, and other autoimmune diseases where B-cells play a pathogenic role. Three forms of pulmonary toxicity described are an ARDS reaction with alveolar hemorrhage, a hypersensitivity reaction and organizing pneumonia. In rare reports, rituximab has caused an ARDS reaction occurring within hours after infusion. In some cases, there has been an association of nonspecific interstitial pneumonitis and usual interstitial pneumonitis. Late-onset of symptoms and the development of organizing pneumonia have been reported. However, the most common clinical presentation of rituximab-related pneumonitis is a subacute presentation accompanied with fever, dyspnea, and hypoxemia. Multiple focal alveolar opacities and ground-glass changes are typically seen. BAL lymphocytosis and a histologic pattern of organizing pneumonia are the most common findings.[146-150]

Interferon

Interferon (INF) alfa-2a and INF alfa-2b are the two commercially available recombinant INFs available in the United States. They are pegylated in order to increase drug's half-life. INF is typically used in conjunction with ribavirin for the treatment of hepatitis C viral infections. INF-related pulmonary toxicities include nonspecific interstitial pneumonia, granulomatosis pneumonitis, organizing pneumonia and bronchospasm. It has been speculated that INF toxicity in at-risk patients is related to an exaggerated Th1 response with the induction of proinflammatory cytokines. Most of the patients recover with drug discontinuation, while others have used systemic corticosteroids and continued with INF therapy.[3,4,151]

Anti-TNF Alfa Drugs

Infliximab, etanercept, and adalimumab are the three commercially available anti-TNF alfa medications approved in the United States. The drugs are commonly used in the treatment of Crohn's disease, psoriasis, rheumatoid arthritis, and ankylosing spondylitis. The most common adverse event associated with these drugs is related to the immunomodulating effect predisposing the patient to infections, including opportunistic pathogens and tuberculosis. Interstitial pneumonitis with pulmonary fibrosis is reported between 0.5% and 0.6% of cases.[4,81-87] A sarcoid-like reaction with anti-TNF alfa therapy has also been reported.[87] The frequency of this reaction has been reported in 0.04% of treated cases with a median time of clinical presentation of 18 months. The most frequent radiographic findings are pulmonary opacities with hilar and mediastinal lymphadenopathy. Noncaseating granulomas from fine-needle aspiration of mediastinal lymph nodes, transbronchial biopsy of lung tissue and skin biopsy have been documented. Improvement was observed in all cases with drug discontinuation with or without systemic corticosteroids.

Rapamycin Analogs

Temsirolimus, a rapamycin analog, is active against renal cell carcinoma, breast cancer, endometrial carcinoma, glioblastoma multiforme, and GI neuroendocrine tumors. It binds with immunophilin FK-506 binding protein-12 and forms a complex that inhibits the protein activity of mTOR. mTOR, a serine kinase, regulates cell growth and apoptosis. Interstitial pneumonitis has been reported in 1–36% of patients. It is a non-dose dependent complication that usually develops between 2 weeks and 16 weeks. Up to 50% of patients with temsirolimus-induced pneumonitis are clinically asymptomatic.[4,152,153]

Everolimus, another rapamycin analog, inhibits mTOR activity. Clinical use of everolimus has been limited to immunosuppression following organ transplantation. Everolimus pneumonitis has been reported in 3% of patients within four weeks of initiation of therapy. All patients, reported in a single series, developed profound hypoxic respiratory failure requiring mechanical ventilation.[154]

Monoclonal Antibodies

Bevacizumab, an antiangiogenic monoclonal antibody, inhibits vascular endothelial growth factor-A. It is currently used in the treatment of metastatic colorectal carcinoma, advanced non-small cell lung cancer (excluding squamous histology), breast cancer, and glioblastoma multiforme. Pulmonary hemorrhage has been reported in 2% of patients with nonsquamous and non-small cell lung cancer.[155-157] Severe pulmonary hemorrhage has been reported in 30% of patients with squamous cell carcinoma. Bevacizumab also increases the risk of deep vein thrombosis and pulmonary embolism.[155-157]

Antineoplastic Agents

Antineoplastic agent-induced pulmonary toxicity is an important contributor to the development of respiratory failure. Although the overall incidence of pulmonary toxicity remains low, more cases are expected with the introduction of newer generation agents as well as establishing new indications for older drugs.[4]

The alkylating agents include chlorozotocin, oxaliplatin, ifosfamide, and temozolomide. Chlorozotocin has activity against islet-cell carcinoma. Several cases of mild interstitial pneumonitis have been reported with this drug.[158,159]

Ifosfamide, an alkylating agent, is used in the treatment of lung cancer, ovarian cancer, sarcomas, and breast cancer. Fatal interstitial pneumonitis have been reported.[160] 4-thioifosfamide is the active metabolite shown to induce methemoglobinemia by depleting red blood cell antioxidant, glutathione, stores in susceptible patients.[161]

Oxaplatin is a recently added alkylating agent used in the treatment of colorectal carcinoma. Interstitial pneumonitis with fibrosis has been reported within 3–6 months of therapy. Fatal pneumonitis occurring within 10 days has also been recognized.[4,162,163] An infusion-related anaphylactic reaction occurs in 1.3% of cases.[164] Eosinophilic pneumonia after oxaliplatin therapy has been reported in a single case report.[165]

Temozolomide is a new generation alkylating agent used in the treatment of anaplastic astrocytoma and metastatic melanoma. Interstitial pneumonitis occurred at a rate of 5% with one patient-related mortality.[166,167]

The cytotoxic antibiotics include doxorubicin, epirubicin, and mitoxantrone. Doxurubicin inhibits topoisomerase II and has activity against many epithelial tumors and sarcomas. Infusion reactions have occurred in 8% of cases.[168] Dyspnea may develop within 1–5 minutes and resolves by stopping the infusion. Several cases of doxorubicin-induced organizing pneumonia have been described.[169,170]

Epiribucin is a cytotoxic antibiotic used in the treatment of lymphoma, breast, ovarian, gastric, and lung carcinoma. Severe pneumonitis can occur within weeks following thoracic radiation. Interstitial pneumonitis occurred in 9% of patients treated with epiribucin in combination with cyclophosphamide and 5-fluorouracil. It is unclear if epiribucin causes direct lung toxicity or simply potentiates the toxicity effects of other drugs or radiation.[4,171]

Mitoxantrone is a newer generation topoisomerase II inhibitor, used primarily in the treatment of metastatic breast cancer. Severe acute pneumonitis has been reported. Both the hypersensitivity and organizing pneumonia-like reaction have been described on pathologic specimens.[172-174]

Piritrexim, a second-generation antimetobolite, is used in the treatment of transitional cell cancer. Pulmonary toxicity is reported in 14% of piritrexim-treated cases.[175] Severe interstitial pneumonitis and respiratory failure have been reported.[176] The respiratory failure was resolved with drug discontinuation. Similar to methotrexate, the presence of pleural effusions or ascites requires complete evacuation prior to piritrexim administration.

Gemcitabine is a nucleoside analog with activity against non-small cell lung cancer and pancreatic adenocarcinoma. Gemcitabine-induced pneumonitis is reported to occur in less than 1% of patients. Three types of gemcitabine-induced pulmonary reactions described are a capillary leak syndrome with pulmonary edema; ARDS; and pulmonary alveolar hemorrhage. Concurrent treatment with other cytotoxic agents, radiation exposure, granulocyte colony-stimulating factor, and pre-existing lung disease are reported risk factors in the development of gemcitabine-related pulmonary toxicity.[4,177-183]

Etoposide and teniposide are podophyllotoxins and inhibitors of topoisomerase II. Etoposide is used in the treatment of small cell lung cancer. A hypersensitivity reaction is the most common presentation for etoposide-induced pulmonary toxicity. Angioedema, cough, bronchospasm, chest pain, and hypotension are the typical findings. Etoposide-induced ARDS has rarely been reported.[184-187] Teniposide is used in the treatment of high-grade astrocytomas. Hypersensitivity reactions occur in 4-7% of patients. The hypersensitivity reaction following teniposide administration is unpredictable and may occur at any treatment cycle.[188]

The topoisomerase-1 inhibitors include irinotecan, topotecan, and exatecan. Irinotecan is used in the treatment of colon cancer and other epithelial tumors. Pneumonitis is dose-dependent with moderate-to-severe pneumonitis occurring in 2-16% of treated patients. Respiratory failure requiring mechanical ventilation may be seen in up to 9% of patients. Fatalities attributed to irinotecan-induced ARDS are seen in approximately 3.5% of cases.[189-192] Topotecan is used in the treatment of small cell lung cancer and metastatic ovarian cancer. Dyspnea is reported in 4% of patients receiving this drug. Cases of ARDS and severe organizing pneumonia resulting in respiratory failure have been reported.[193,194] A new topoisomerase I inhibitor, exatecan, is being studied in the treatment of numerous neoplasms. In a phase-II study, mild-to-moderate dyspnea developed in 36% of patients.[195]

The taxanes, paclitaxel, and docetaxel are used in the treatment of breast, ovarian, and lung carcinomas. Docetaxel-induced pneumonitis occurs in 7-26% of patients, while paclitaxel-induced pneumonitis occurs in 0.7-12%. Dyspnea, cough, and bilateral parenchymal infiltrates develop in between 7 days and 90 days after taxane exposure. Reported risk factors are weekly or biweekly infusions and concurrent treatment with gemcitabine and irinotecan. Mild cases of pneumonitis tend to resolve with or without moderate doses of corticosteroids. Mild pneumonitis is not a contraindication to subsequent taxane administration. Severe taxane-induced pneumonitis and death have been described. Infusion-related reactions with bronchospasm, cough, and hypotension can occur.[4,196-203]

Thalidomide has been approved for the treatment of multiple myeloma and is being investigated in the treatment of other neoplastic and non-neoplastic diseases.[204] Thalidomide-related dyspnea has been reported in approximately 50% of cases.[205] Opportunistic infections have been described in leukopenic patients receiving thalidomide.[206] Thalidomide increases the risk for deep vein thrombosis and venous thromboembolism; however, prophylactic administration of anticoagulant therapy has not been suggested.[207] Interstitial fibrosis, organizing pneumonia, and lymphocytic alveolitis have been reported.[4,208,209]

REFERENCES

1. Rosenow EC III. The spectrum of drug-induced pulmonary disease. *Ann Intern Med.* 1972;77:977-91.
2. Pneumotox online: the drug-induced lung diseases. www.pneumotox.com. Last update: June 16, 2010.
3. Bauman KA, Chan KM. Drug-induced lung disease. Pulmonary, Critical Care, and Sleep Update. Northbrook, Illinois: American College of Chest Physicians; 2010.
4. Vahid B, Marik PE. Pulmonary complications of novel antineoplastic agents for solid tumors. *Chest.* 2008;133:528-38.
5. Barrera P, Laan RF, van Riel PL, et al. Methotrexate-related pulmonary complications in rheumatoid arthritis. *Ann Rheum Dis.* 1994;53:434-9.
6. Alarcon GS, Kremer JM, Macaluso M, et al. Risk factors for methotrexate-induced lung injury in patients with rheumatoid arthritis. *Ann Intern Med.* 1997;127:356-64.
7. Delaunois LM. Mechanisms in pulmonary toxicology. *Clin Chest Med.* 2004;25:1-14.
8. Lindell RM, Hartman TE. Chest imaging in iatrogenic respiratory disease. *Clin Chest Med.* 2004;25:15-24.
9. Flieder DB, Travis WD. Pathologic characteristics of drug-induced lung disease. *Clin Chest Med.* 2004;25:37-45.
10. Rossi SE, Erasmus JJ, McAdams HP, et al. Pulmonary drug toxicity: radiologic and pathologic manifestations. *Radiographics.* 2000;20:1245-59.
11. Park JS, Lee KS, Kim JS, et al. Nonspecific interstitial pneumonia with fibrosis: radiographic and CT findings in seven patients. *Radiology.* 1995;195:645-8.
12. Johkoh T, Muller NL, Cartier Y, et al. Idiopathic interstitial pneumonias: diagnostic accuracy of thin-section CT in 129 patients. *Radiology.* 1999;211:555-60.
13. Nishiyama O, Kondoh Y, Taniguchi H, et al. Serial high resolution CT findings in nonspecific interstitial pneumonia/fibrosis. *J Comput Assist Tomogr.* 2000;24:41-6.
14. Kuhlman JE, Teigen C, Ren H, et al. Amiodarone pulmonary toxicity: CT findings in symptomatic patients. *Radiology.* 1990;177:121-5.
15. Cooper JA, White DA, Matthay RA. Drug-induced pulmonary disease. Part 1: cytotoxic drugs. *Am Rev Respir Dis.* 1986;133:321-40.
16. Holoye PY, Jenkins DE, Greenberg SD. Pulmonary toxicity of long-term administration of BCNU. *Cancer Treat Rep.* 1976;60:1691-4.
17. Muller NL, Guerry-force ML, Staples CA, et al. Differential diagnosis of bronchiolitis obliterans with organizing pneumonia and usual interstitial pneumonia: clinical, functional, and radiologic findings. *Radiology.* 1987;162:151-6.
18. Grenier P, Chevret S, Beigelman C, et al. Chronic diffuse infiltrative lung disease: determination of the diagnostic value of clinical data, chest radiography, and CT and Bayesian analysis. *Radiology.* 1994;191:383-90.
19. Padley SP, Adler B, Hansell DM, et al. High-resolution computed tomography of drug-induced lung disease. *Clin Radiol Oct.* 1992;6:52-61.
20. Cooper JA, White DA, Matthay RA. Drug-induced pulmonary disease. Part 2: noncytotoxic drugs. *Am Rev Respir Dis.* 1986;133:488-505.
21. Small JH, Flower CD, Traill ZC, et al. Air-trapping in extrinsic allergic alveolitis on computed tomography. *Clin Radiol.* 1996;51:684-8.
22. Hansell DM, Wells AU, Padley SP, et al. Hypersensitivity pneumonitis: correlation of individual CT patterns with functional abnormalities. *Radiology.* 1996;199:123-8.

23. Flores-Franco RA, Luevano-Flores E, Gaston-Ramirez C. Sirolimus-associated desquamative interstitial pneumonia. *Respiration.* 2007;74:237-8.

24. Argiriadi PA, Mendelson DS. High resolution computed tomography in idiopathic interstitial pneumonias. *Mt Sinai J Med.* 2009;76:37-52.

25. Kidney JC, O'Halloran D J, FitzGerald MX. Captopril and lymphocytic alveolitis. *Br Med J.* 1989;299:981.

26. Munn NJ, Baughman RP, Ploysongsang Y, Wirman JA, Bullock WE. Bronchoalveolar lavage in acute drug-hypersensitivity pneumonitis probably caused by phenytoin. *South Med J.* 1984;77:1594-6.

27. Kadikoy H, Paolini M, Achkar K, et al. Pulmonary alveolar proteinosis in a kidney transplant: a rare complication of sirolimus. *Nephrol Dial Transplant.* 2010;25:2795-8.

28. Aquino SL, Webb WR, Golden J. Bronchiolitis obliterans associated with rheumatoid arthritis: findings on HRCT and dynamic expiratory CT. *J Comput Assist Tomogr.* 1994; 18:555-8.

29. McLoud TC, Epler GR, Colby TV, et al. Bronchiolitis obliterans. *Radiology.* 1986;159:1-8.

30. Garg K, Lynch DA, Newell JD, et al. Proliferative and constrictive bronchiolitis: classification and radiologic features. *Am J Roentgenol.* 1994;162:803-8.

31. Rosenow III EC, Myers JL, Swensen SJ, et al. Drug-induced pulmonary disease. An update. *Chest.* 1992;102:239-50.

32. Akira M, Yamamoto S, Sakatani M. Bronchiolitis obliterans organizing pneumonia manifesting as multiple pulmonary nodules or masses. *Am J Roentgenol.* 1998;170:291-5.

33. Muller NL, Staples CA, Miller RR. Bronchiolitis obliterans organizing pneumonia: CT features in 14 patients. *Am J Roentgenol.* 1990;154:983-7.

34. Wesselius LJ. Pulmonary complications of cancer therapy. *Compr Ther.* 1999;25:272-5.

35. Reed CR, Glauser FL. Drug-induced noncardiogenic pulmonary edema. *Chest.* 1991; 100:1120-4.

36. Gluecker T, Capasso P, Schnyder P, et al. Clinical and radiographic features of pulmonary edema. *Radiographics.* 1999;19:1507-31.

37. Storto ML, Kee ST, Golden JA, et al. Hydrostatic pulmonary edema: high-resolution CT findings. *Am J Roentgenol.* 1995;165:817-20.

38. Schwarz MI, Fontenot A. Drug-induced diffuse alveolar hemorrhage syndromes and vasculitis. *Clin Chest Med.* 2004;25:133-40.

39. Schwarz MI, Brown KK. Small vessel vasculitis of the lung. *Thorax.* 2000;55:502-10.

40. Stankus SJ, Johnson NT. Propylthiouracil-induced hypersensitivity vasculitis presenting as respiratory failure. *Chest.* 1992;102:1595-6.

41. Yermakov VM, Hitti IF, Sutton AL. Necrotizing vasculitis associated with diphenyl-hydantoin: two fatal cases. *Hum Pathol.* 1983;14:182-4.

42. Frankel SR, Eardley A, Lauwers G, et al. The "retinoic acid syndrome" in acute promyelocytic leukemia. *Ann Intern Med.* 1992;117:292-6.

43. Dhillion SS, Singh D, Doe N, et al. Diffuse alveolar hemorrhage and pulmonary capillaritis due to propylthiouracil. *Chest.* 1999;116:1485-8.

44. D'Cruz D, Chesser AM, Lightowler C, et al. Antineutrophil cytoplasmic antibody-positive cresentic glomerulonephritis assoicated with anti-thyroid drug treatments. *Br J Rheumatol.* 1995;34:1090-1.

45. Ohtsuka M, Yamashita Y, Doi M, et al. Propylthiouracil-induced alveolar hemorrhage associated with antinuclear cytoplasmic antibody. *Eur Respir J.* 1997;10:1405-7.

46. Jones BF, Major GA. Crescentic glomerulonephritis in a patient taking penicillamine associated with antineutrophil cytoplasmic antibody. *Clin Nephrol.* 1992;38:293.

47. Mathieson PW, Peat DS, Short A, et al. Coexistent membranous nephropathy and ANCA-positive crescentic glomerulonephritis in association with penicillamine. *Nephrol Dial Transplant.* 1996;11:863-6.

48. Gaskin G, Thompson EM, Pusey CD. Goodpasture-like syndrome associated with anti-myeloperoxidase antibodies following penicillamine treatment. *Nephrol Dial Transplant.* 1995;10:1925-8.

49. Torra R, Poch E, Torras A, et al. Pulmonary hemorrhage as a clinical manifestation of hemolytic-uremic syndrome assoicated with mitomycin C therapy. *Chemotherapy.* 1993;39:453-6.

50. Hackman RC, Madtes DK, Petersen FB, et al. Pulmonary veno-occulsive disease following bone marrow transplantation. *Transplantation.* 1989;47:989-92.

51. Williams LM, Fussell S, Veith RQ, et al. Pulmonary veno-occulsive disease in an adult following bone marrow transplantation. Case report and review of the literature. *Chest.* 1996;109:1388-91.

52. Mulder PO, Meinesz AF, de Vries EG, et al. Diffuse alveolar hemorrhage in autologous bone marrow transplant recipients. *Am J Med.* 1991;90:278-81.

53. Bucknall CE, Adamson MR, Banham SW. Nonfatal pulmonary hemorrhage associated with nitrofurantoin. *Thorax.* 1987;42:475-6.

54. Garcia R, Garcia BF, Puras Gil AM. Pulmonary hemorrhage and antiglomerular basement membrane antibody-mediated glomerulonephritis after exposure to smoked cocaine (crack): a case report and review of the literature. *Pathol Int.* 1997;47:692-7.

55. Bailey ME, Fraire AE, Greenberg SD, et al. Pulmonary histopathology in cocaine abusers. *Hum Pathol.* 1994;25:203-7.

56. Barnett VT, Bergmann F, Humphrey H, et al. Diffuse alveolar hemorrhage secondary to superwarfarin ingestion. *Chest.* 1992;102:1301-2.

57. Kalra S, Bell MR, Rihal CS. Alveolar hemorrhage as a complication of treatment with abciximab. *Chest.* 2001;120:126-31.

58. Sleiman C, Raffy O, Roué C, et al. Fatal pulmonary hemorrhage during high-dose valproate monotherapy. *Chest.* 2000;117:613.

59. Kilaru PK, Schweiger MJ, Kozman HA, et al. Diffuse alveolar hemorrhage after clopidro-grel use. *J Invasive Cardiol.* 2001;13:535-7.

60. Gopalakrishnan D, Tioran T, Emanuel C, et al. Diffuse pulmonary hemorrhage complicating thrombolytic therapy for acute myocardial infarction. *Clin Cardiol.* 1997;20:298-300.

61. Masip J, Vecilla F, Paez J. Diffuse pulmonary hemorrhage after fibrinolytic therapy for acute myocardial infarction. *Int J Cardiol.* 1998;63:95-7.

62. Allen JN. Drug-induced eosinophilic lung disease. *Clin Chest Med.* 2004;25:77-88.

63. Allen JN, Davis WB. State of the art: the eosinophilic lung dieases. *Am J Respir Crit Care Med.* 1994;150:1423-38.

64. Darmanata JI, van Zandwijk N, Duren DR, et al. Amiodarone pneumonitis: three further cases with a review of published reports. *Thorax.* 1984;39:57-64.

65. Jennings CA, Deveikis J, Azumi N, et al. Eosinophilic pneumonia associated with reaction to radiographic contrast medium. *South Med J.* 1991;87:92-5.

66. Mahatma M, Haponik EF, Nelson S, et al. Phenytoin-induced acute respiratory failure with pulmonary eosinophilia. *Am J Med.* 1989;87:93-4.

67. White DA, Kris MG, Stover DE. Bronchoalveolar lavage cell populations in bleomycin lung toxicity. *Thorax.* 1987;42:551-2.

68. Akoun GM, Cadranel JL, Milleron GJ, et al. Bronchoalveolar lavage cell data in 19 patients with drug-associated pneumonitis (except amiodarone). *Chest.* 1991;99:98-104.

69. Kaufman LD, Seidman RJ, Gruber BL. L-tryptophan-associated eosinophilic perimyositis, neuritis, and fasciitis. A clinicopathologic and laboratory study of 25 patients. *Medicine.* 1990;69:187-99.

70. Sitbon O, Bidel N, Dussopt C, et al. Minocycline-induced eosinophilic pneumonitis: an analysis in 5 patients. *Am Rev Respir Dis.* 1993;147:A76.

71. Davies D, Lloyd-Jones J. Pulmonary eosinophilia caused by penicillamine. *Thorax.* 1980; 35:957-8.

72. Middleton K, Santella R, Couser JI Jr. Eosinophilic pleuritis due to propylthiouracil. *Chest.* 1993;103:955-6.

73. Fiegenberg DS, Weiss H, Kirshman H. Migratory pneumonia with eosinophilia associated with sulfamide administration. *Arch Intern Med.* 1967;120:85-9.

74. Wilson IC, Gambill JM, Sandifer MG. Loeffler's syndrome occurring during imipramine therapy. *Am J Psychiatry.* 1963;119:892-3.

75. Riechlin S, Loveless MH, Kane EG. Loeffler's syndrome following penicillin therapy. *Ann Intern Med.* 1953;38:113-20.

76. Ecker MD, Jay B, Keohane MF. Procarbazine lung. *Am J Roentgenol.* 1978;131:527-8.

77. Knoell DL, Lucas J, Allen JN. Churg-Strauss syndrome associated with zafirlukast. *Chest.* 1998;114:332-4.

78. Wechsler ME, Garpestad E, Flier SR, et al. Pulmonary infiltrates, eosinophilia, and cardiomyopathy following corticosteroid withdrawal in patients with asthma receiving zafirlukast. *JAMA.* 1998;279:455-7.

79. Guilpain P, Viallard JF, Lagarde P, et al. Churg-Strauss syndrome in two patients receiving montelukast. *Rheumatol.* 2002;41:535-9.

80. Gupta RC, Lavengood R Jr, Smith JP. Miliary tuberculosis due to intravesical bacillus Calmette-Guerin therapy. *Chest.* 1988;94(6):296-8.

81. Furst DE, Wallis R, Broder M, Beenhouwer DO. Tumor necrosis factor antagonists: different kinetics and/or mechanisms of action may explain differences in the risk for developing granulomatous infection. *Semin Arthritis Rheum.* 2006;36:159-67.

82. Saag KG, Teng GG, Patkar NM, et al. American College of Rheumatology 2008 recommendations for the use of nonbiologic and biologic disease-modifying antirheumatic drugs in rheumatoid arthritis. *Arthritis Rheum.* 2008;59:762-84.

83. Ostör AJ, Chilvers ER, Somerville MF, et al. Pulmonary complications of infliximab therapy in patients with rheumatoid arthritis. *J Rheumatol.* 2006;33:622-8.

84. Huggett MT, Armstrong R. Adalimumab-associated pulmonary fibrosis. *Rheumatology.* 2006;45:1312-3.

85. Takeuchi T, Tatsuki Y, Nogami Y, et al. Postmarketing surveillance of the safety profile of infliximab in 5000 Japanese patients with rheumatoid arthritis. *Ann Rheum Dis.* 2008;67:189-94.

86. Lindsay K, Melsom R, Jacob BK, Mestry N. Acute progression of interstitial lung disease: a complication of etanercept particularly in the presence of rheumatoid lung and methotrexate treatment. *Rheumatology.* 2006;45:1048-9.

87. Daïen CI, Monnier A, Claudepierre P, et al. Sarcoid-like granulomatosis in patients treated with tumor necrosis factor blockers: 10 cases. *Rheumatology.* 2009;48:883-6.

88. Dicpinigaitis PV. Angiotensin-converting enzyme inhibitor-induced cough: ACCP evidence-based clinical practice guidelines. *Chest.* 2006;129:169S-73.

89. Isralli ZH, Hall WD. Cough and angioneurotic edema associated with angiotensin-converting enzyme inhibitor therapy: a review of the literature and pathophysiology. *Ann Intern Med.* 1992;117:234-42.

90. Irwin RS, Baumann MH, Bolser DC, et al. Diagnosis and management of cough executive summary: ACCP evidence-based clinical practice guidelines. *Chest.* 2006;129:1-23S.

91. Agarwal A, Azim A, Ambesh S, et al. Salbutamol, beclomethasone or sodium chromoglycate suppress coughing induced by iv fentanyl. *Can J Anaesth.* 2003;50:297-300.

92. Tweed WA, Dakin D. Explosive coughing after bolus fentanyl injection. *Anesth Analg.* 2001;92:1442-3.

93. Schnabel A, Dalhoff K, Bauerfeind S, et al. Sustained cough in methotrexate therapy for rheumatoid arthritis. *Clin Rheumatol.* 1996;15:277-82.

94. Bennett-Guerrero E, Young CC. Bronchospasm after intravenous adenosine administration. *Anesth Analg.* 1994;79:386-8.

95. Plaza V, Serrano J, Picado C, et al. Frequency and clinical characteristics of rapid- onset of fatal and near-fatal asthma. *Eur Respir J.* 2002;19:846-52.

96. Toronto Aerosolized Pentamidine Study (TAPS) Group. Acute pulmonary effects of aerosolized pentamidine: a randomized controlled study. *Chest.* 1990;98:907-10.

97. Huggins JT, Sahn SA. Drug-induced pleural disease. *Clin Chest Med.* 2004;25:141-53.

98. Antony VB. Drug-induced pleural disease. *Clin Chest Med.* 1998;19:331-40.

99. Morelock SY, Sahn SA. Drugs and the pleura. *Chest.* 1999;116:212-21.

100. Goldblatt M, Huggins JT, Doelken P, et al. Dasatinib-induced pleural effusions: a lymphatic network disorder? *Am J Med Sci.* 2009;338:414-7.

101. Hoffman BJ. Sensitivity of sulfadiazine resembling acute disseminated lupus erythematosus. *Arch Dermatol Syph.* 1945;51:190-2.

102. Yung YL, Richardson BC. Drug-induced lupus. *Rheum Dis Clin N Am.* 1994;20:61-85.

103. Good JT, King TE, Antony VB, et al. Lupus pleuritis: clinical features and pleural fluid characteristics with special reference to pleural fluid antinuclear antibody titers. *Chest.* 1983;84:714-5.

104. Cockerill FR III, Wilson WR, Carpenter H, et al. Open lung biopsy in immunocompromised patients. *Arch Intern Med.* 1985;145:1398-404.

105. Costabel U, Uzalan E, Guzman J. Bronchoalveolar lavage in drug-induced lung disease. *Clin Chest Med.* 2004;25:25-35.

106. Camus P, Martin III WJ, Rosenow EC. Amiodarone pulmonary toxicity. *Clin Chest Med.* 2004;25:65-75.

107. McGovern B, Garan H, Kelly E, et al. Adverse reactions during treatment with amiodarone. *Br Med J* (Clin Res Ed). 1983;287:175-80.

108. Dean PJ, Groshart KD, Porterfield JG, et al. Amiodarone-associated pulmonary toxicity. A clinical and pathologic study of eleven cases. *Am J Clin Pathol.* 1987;87:7-13.

109. Cox G, Johnson J, Kinnear WJM, et al. Amiodarone and the lung: wide variations in clinical practice. *Respir Med.* 2000;94:1130-1.

110. Morady F, Sauve MJ, Malone P, et al. Long-term efficacy and toxicity of high-dose amiodarone therapy for ventricular tachycardia or ventricular fibrillation. *Am J Cardiol.* 1983;52:975-9.

111. Kay GN, Epstein AE, Kirklin JK, et al. Fatal postoperative amiodarone pulmonary toxicity. *Am J Cardiol.* 1988;62:490-2.

112. Van Mieghem W, Coolen L, Malysse I, et al. Amiodarone and the development of ARDS after lung surgery. *Chest.* 1994;105:1642-5.

113. Handschin AE, Lardinosis D, Schneiter D, et al. Acute amiodarone-induced pulmonary toxicity following lung resection. *Respiration.* 2003;70:310-2.

114. Kharabsheh S, Abendroth CS, Kozak M. Fatal pulmonary toxicity occurring within two weeks of initiation of amiodarone. *Am J Cardiol.* 2002;89:896-8.

115. Wood DL, Osborn MJ, Rooke J, et al. Amiodarone pulmonary toxicity: report of two cases associated with rapidly progressive fatal adult respiratory distress syndrome after pulmonary angiography. *Mayo Clin Proc.* 1985;60:601-3.

116. Lee-Chiong TL, Matthay RA. Drug-induced pulmonary edema and acute respiratory distress syndrome. *Clin Chest Med.* 2004;25:95-104.

117. Mendez JL, Nadrous HF, Hartman TE, et al. Chronic nitrofurantoin-induced lung disease. *Mayo Clin Proc.* 2005;80:1298-302.

118. Rosenow EC, DeRemee RA, Dines DE. Chronic nitrofurantoin pulmonary reaction. Report of 5 cases. *N Engl J Med.* 1968;279:1258-62.

119. Cohen AJ, King TE, Downey GP. Rapidly progressive bronchiolitis obliterans with organizing pneumonia. *Am J Respir Crit Care Med.* 1994;149:1670-5.

120. Cameron RJ, Kolbe J, Wilsher ML, et al. Bronchiolitis obliterans organizing pneumonia associated with the use of nitrofurantoin. *Thorax.* 2000;55:249-51.

121. Fawcett IW, Ibrahim NB. BOOP associated with nitrofurantoin. *Thorax.* 2001;56:161.

122. Fenton ME, Kanthan R, Cockcroft DW. Nitrofurnatoin-associated bronchiolitis obliterans organizing pneumonia: Report of a case. *Can Respir J.* 2008;15:311-2.

123. Popovsky MA, Abel MD, Moore SB. Transfusion-related acute lung injury associated with passive transfer of antileukocyte antibodies. *Am Rev Respir Dis.* 1983;128:185-9.

124. Kopko PM, Popovsky MA. Pulmonary injury from transfusion-related acute lung injury. *Clin Chest Med.* 2004;25:105-11.

125. Looney MR, Gilliss BM, Matthay MA. Pathophysiology of transfusion-related acute lung injury. *Curr Opin Hematol.* 2010;17:418-23.

126. Corwin HL, Gettinger A, Pearl RG, et al. The CRIT Study: anemia and blood transfusions in the critically ill—current clinical practice in the United States. *Crit Care Med.* 2004; 32:39-52.

127. Vincent JL, Baron JF, Reinhart K, et al. Anemia and blood transfusion in critically ill patients. *JAMA.* 2002;288:1499-507.

128. Benson AB, Austin GL, Berg M, et al. Transfusion-related acute lung injury in ICU patients admitted with gastrointestinal bleeding. *Intensive Care Med.* 2010.

129. Kelher MR, Masuno T, Moore EE, et al. Plasma from stored packed red blood cells and MHC Class 1 antibodies causes acute lung injury in a 2-event *in vivo* rat model. *Blood.* 2009;113:2079-87.

130. Sachs UJ, Hattar K, Weissmann N, et al. Antibody-induced neutrophil activation as a trigger for transfusion-related acute lung injury in an *ex vivo* rat lung model. *Blood.* 2006;107:1217-9.

131. Silliman CC, Paterson AJ, Dickey WO, et al. The association of biologically active lipids with the development of transfusion-related acute lung injury: a retrospective study. *Transfusion.* 1997;37:719-26.

132. Silliman CC, Voelkel NF, Allard JD, et al. Plasma and lipids from stored packed red blood cells cause acute lung injury in an animal model. *J Clin Invest.* 1998;101:1458-67.

133. Silliman CC, Bjornsen AJ, Wyman TH, et al. Plasma and lipids from stored platelets cause acute lung injury in an animal model. *Transfusion.* 2003;43:633-40.

134. Triulzi DJ, Kleinman S, Kakaiya RM, et al. The effect of previous pregnancy and transfusion on HLA alloimmunization in blood donors: implications for a transfusion-related acute lung injury risk reduction strategy. *Transfusion.* 2009;49:1825-35.

135. Densmore TL, Goodnough LT, Ali S, et al. Prevalence of HLA sensitization in female apheresis donors. *Transfusion.* 1999;39:103-6.

136. Chapman CE, Stainsby D, Jones H, et al. Ten years of hemovigilance reports of transfusion-related acute lung injury in the United Kingdom and the impact of preferential use of male donors. *Transfusion.* 2009;49:440-52.

137. Shih YN, Chiu CH, Tsai CM, et al. Interstitial pneumonia during gefitinib treatment on non-small cell lung cancer. *J Chin Med Assoc.* 2005;68:183-6.

138. Park K, Goto K. A review of the benefit-risk profile of gefitinib in Asian patients with advanced non-small cell lung cancer. *Curr Med Res Opin.* 2006;22:561-73.

139. Ando M, Okamoto I, Yamamoto N, et al. Predictive factors for interstitial lung disease, antitumor responses, and survival in non-small cell lung cancer patients treated with gefitinib. *J Clin Oncol.* 2006;24:2549-56.

140. Chou CL, Ko HW, Wang CW, et al. Erlotinib-associated near fatal interstitial pneumonitis in a patient with relapsed lung adenocarcinoma. *Chang Gung Med.* 2010;33:100-4.

141. Peters CW, Loneragan R, Clarke S. Cetuximab-associated pulmonary toxicity. *Clin Colorectal Cancer.* 2009;8:118-20.

142. Ohnishi K, Sakai F, Kudoh S, et al. Twenty-seven cases of drug-induced interstitial lung disease associated with imatinib. *Leukemia.* 2006;20:1162-4.

143. Ma CX, Hobday TJ, Jett JR. Imatinib mesylate-induced interstitial pneumonitis. *Mayo Clin Proc.* 2003;78:1578-9.

144. Grimison P, Goldstein D, Schneeweiss J, et al. Corticosteroid-responsive interstitial pneumonitis related to imatinib mesylate with successful rechallenge, and potential causative mechanisms. *Intern Med J.* 2005;35:136-7.

145. Lin JT, Yeh KT, Fang HY, et al. Fulminant, but reversible interstitial pneumonitis associated with imatinib mesylate. *Leuk Lymphoma.* 2006;47:1693-5.

146. Wu SJ, Chou WC, Ko BS, et al. Severe pulmonary complications after initial treatment with rituximab for the Asian-variant of intravascular lymphoma. *Hematologica.* 2007;92:141-2.

147. Burton C, Kaczmarski R, Jan-Mohamed R. Interstitial pneumonitis related to rituximab therapy. *N Engl J Med.* 2003;348:2690-1.

148. Wagner SA, Mehta AC, Laber DA. Rituximab-induced interstitial lung disease. *Am J Hematol.* 2007;82:916-9.

149. Heresi GA, Farver CF, Stoller JK. Intersititial pneumonitis and alveolar hemorrhage complicating use of rituximab. Case report and review of the literature. *Respiration.* 2008;76:449-53.

150. Tonelli AR, Lottenberg R, Allan RW, et al. Rituximab-induced hypersensitivity pneumonitis. *Respiration.* 2009;78:225-9.

151. Nakamura F, Andoh A, Minamiguchi H, et al. A case of interstitial pneumonitis associated with natural alfa-interferon therapy for myelofibrosis. *Acta Hematol.* 1997;97:222-4.

152. Atkins MB, Hidalgo M, Stadler WM, et al. Randomized phase II study of multiple dose levels of CCI-779, a novel mammalian target of rapamycin kinase inhibitor, in patients with advanced refractory renal cell carcinoma. *J Clin Oncol.* 2004;22:909-18.

153. Duran I, Siu LL, Oza AM, et al. Characterization of the lung toxicity of the cell cycle inhibitor temisirolimus. *Eur J Cancer.* 2006;42:1875-80.

154. Rothenburger M, Teerling E, Bruch C, et al. Calcineurin inhibitor-free immunosuppression using everolimus (Certican) in maintenance heart transplant recipients: 6 months' follow-up. *J Heart Lung Transplant.* 2007;26:250-57

155. Sandler A, Gray R, Perry MC, et al. Paclitaxel-carboplatin alone or with bevacizumab for non-small-cell lung cancer. *N Engl J Med.* 2006;355:2542-50.

156. Herbst RS, Sandler AB. Non-small cell lung cancer and antiangiogenic therapy: what can be expected of bevacizumab? *Oncologist.* 2004;9:19-26.

157. Johnson DH, Fehrenbacher L, Novotny WF, et al. Randomized phase II trial comparing bevacizumab plus carboplatin and paclitaxel with carboplatin and paclitaxel alone in previously untreated locally advanced or metastatic non-small-cell lung cancer. *J Clin Oncol*. 2004;22:2184-91.

158. Sordillo EM, Sordillo PP, Stover D, et al. Chlorozotocin (DCNU)-induced pulmonary toxicity. *Cancer Clin Trials*. 1981;4:397-9.

159. Geodert JJ, Smith FP, Tsou E, et al. Combination chemotherapy pneumonitis: a case report of possible synergistic toxicity. *Pediatr Oncol*. 1983;11:116-8.

160. Baker WJ, Fistel SJ, Jones RV, et al. Interstitial pneumonitis associated with ifosfamide therapy. *Cancer*. 1990;65:2217-21.

161. Hadjiliadis D, Govert JA. Methemoglobinemia after infusion of ifosfamide chemotherapy. *Chest*. 2000;118:1208-10.

162. Pasetto LM, Monfardini S. Is acute dyspnea related to oxaliplatin administration? *World J Gastroenterol*. 2006;12:5907-8.

163. Yague XH, Soy E, Merino BQ, et al. Interstitial pneumonitis after oxaliplatin treatment in colorectal cancer. *Clin Transl Oncol*. 2005;7:515-7.

164. Gagnadoux F, Roiron C, Carrie E, et al. Eosinophilic lung disease under chemotherapy with oxaliplatin for colorectal cancer. *Am J Clin Oncol*. 2002;25:388-90.

165. Lee MY, Yang MH, Liu JH, et al. Severe anaphylactic reactions in patients receiving oxalipatin therapy: a rare but potentially fatal complication. *Support Care Cancer*. 2007; 15:89-93.

166. Abrey LE, Oslon JD, Raizer JJ, et al. A phase II trial of temozolomide for patients with recurrent or progressive brain metastasis. *J Neurooncol*. 2001;53:259-65.

167. Brandwein JM, Yang L, Schimmer AD, et al. A phase II study of temozolomide therapy for poor-risk patients aged ≥ 60 years with acute myeloid leukemia: low levels of MGMT predict for response. *Leukemia*. 2007;21:821-4.

168. Skubitz KM, Skubitz AP. Mechanism of transient dyspnea induced by pegylated liposomal doxorubicin (Doxil). *Anticancer Drugs*. 1998;9:45-50.

169. Tsao YT, Dai MS, Chang H, et al. Bronchiolitis obliterans organizing pneumonia presenting as hemoptysis in a patient of Hodgkin's lymphoma undergoing chemotherapy. *J Med Sci*. 2006;26:115-8.

170. Jacobs C, Slade M, Lavery B. Doxorubicin and BOOP. A possible near fatal association. *Clin Oncol*. 2002;14:262.

171. Dang CT, D'Andrea GM, Moynahan ME, et al. Phase II study of feasibility of dose-dense FEC followed by alternating weekly taxanes in high-risk, four or more node-positive breast cancer. *Clin Cancer Res*. 2004;10:5754-61.

172. Tomlinson J, Tighe M, Johnson S, et al. Interstitial pneumonitis following mitozantrone, chlorambucil and prednisolone (MCP) chemotherapy. *Clin Oncol*. 1999;11:184-6.

173. Quigley M, Brada M, Heron C, et al. Severe lung toxicity with a weekly low dose chemotherapy regimen in patients with non-Hodgkin's lymphoma. *Hematol Oncol*. 1988;6:319-24.

174. Matsukawa Y, Takeuchi J, Aiso M, et al. Interstitial pneumonitis possibly due to mitoxantrone. *Acta Haematol*. 1993;90:155-8.

175. Roth BJ, Manola J, Dreicer R, et al. Piritrexim in advanced, refractory carcinoma of the urothelium (E3896): a phase II trial of the Eastern Cooperative Oncology Group. *Invest New Drugs*. 2002;20:425-9.

176. de Wit R, Verweij J, Slingerland R, et al. Piritrexim-induced pulmonary toxicity. *Am J Clin Oncol*. 1993;16:146-8.

177. Briasoulis E, Pavlidis N. Noncardiogenic pulmonary edema: an unusual and serious complication of anticancer therapy. *Oncologist.* 2001;6:153-61.

178. Roychowdhury DF, Cassidy CA, Peterson P, et al. A report on serious pulmonary toxicity associated with gemcitabine-based therapy. *Invest New Drugs.* 2002;20:311-5.

179. Gupta N, Ahmed I, Steinberg H, et al. Gemcitabine-induced pulmonary toxicity: case report and review of the literature. *Am J Clin Oncol.* 2002;25:96-100.

180. Marruchella A, Fiorenzano G, Merizzi A, et al. Diffuse alveolar damage in a patient treated with gemcitabine. *Eur Respir J.* 1998;11:504-6.

181. Pavlaski N, Bell DR, Millward MJ, et al. Fatal pulmonary toxicity resulting from treatment with gemcitabine. *Cancer.* 1997;80:286-91.

182. Carron PL, Cousin L, Caps T, et al. Gemcitabine-associated diffuse alveolar damage. *Intensive Care Med.* 2001;27:1554.

183. Vander Els NJ, Miller V. Successful treatment of gemcitabine toxicity with a brief course of oral corticosteroid therapy. *Chest.* 1998;114:1779-81.

184. Siderov J, Prasad P, De Boer R, et al. Safe administration of etoposide phosphate after hypersensitivity reaction to intravenous etoposide. *Br J Cancer.* 2002;86:12-3.

185. Dajczman E, Srolovitz H, Kreisman H, et al. Fatal pulmonary toxicity following oral etoposide therapy. *Lung Cancer.* 1995;12:81-6.

186. Gurjal A, An T, Valdivieso M, et al. Etoposide-induced pulmonary toxicity. *Lung Cancer.* 1999;26:109-12.

187. Zimmerman MS, Ruckdeschel JC, Hussain M. Chemotherapy induced interstitial pneumonitis during treatment of small cell anaplastic lung cancer. *J Clin Oncol.* 1984;2:396-405.

188. O'Dwyer PJ, King SA, Fortner CL, et al. Hypersensitivity reactions to teniposide (VM-26): an analysis. *J Clin Oncol.* 1986;8:1262-9.

189. Rocha-Lima CM, Herndon JE II, Lee ME, et al. Phase II trial of irinotecan/gemcitabine as second-line therapy for relapsed and refractory small-cell lung cancer: Cancer and Leukemia Group B Study 39902. *Ann Oncol.* 2007;18:331-7.

190. Kaneda H, Kurata T, Tamura K, et al. A phase I study of irinotecan in combination with amrubicin for advanced lung cancer patients. *Anticancer Res.* 2006;26:2479-85.

191. Klautke G, Fahndrich S, Semrau S, et al. Simultaneous chemoradiotherapy with irinotecan and cisplatin in limited disease small cell lung cancer: a phase I study. *Lung Cancer.* 2006;53:183-8.

192. Madarnas Y, Webster P, Shorter AM, et al. Irinotecan-associated pulmonary toxicity. *Anticancer Drugs.* 2000;11:709-13.

193. O'Brien ME, Ciuleanu TE, Tsekov H, et al. Phase III trial comparing supportive care alone with supportive care with oral topotecan in patients with relapsed small-cell lung cancer. *J Clin Oncol.* 2006;24:5441-7.

194. Pfisterer J, Weber B, Reuss A, et al. Randomized phase III trial of topotecan following carboplatin and paclitaxel in first-line treatment of advanced ovarian cancer: a Gynecologic Cancer Intergoup Trial of the AGO-OVAR and GINECO. *J Natl Cancer Inst.* 2006;98:1036-45.

195. Reichardt P, Nielsen OS, Bauer S, et al. Exatecan in pretreated adult patients with advanced soft tissue sarcoma: results of a phase II-study of the EORTC Soft Tissue and Bone Sarcoma Group. *Eur J Cancer.* 2007;43:1017-22.

196. Shitara K, Ishii E, Kondo M, et al. Suspected paclitaxel-linduced pneumonitis. *Gastric Cancer.* 2006;9:325-8.

197. Suzaki N, Hiraki A, Takigawa N, et al. Severe interstitial pneumonia induced by paclitaxel in a patient with adenocarcinoma of the lung. *Acta Med Okayama*. 2006;60:295-8.

198. Ostoros G, Pretz A, Fillinger J, et al. Fatal pulmonary fibrosis induced by paclitaxel: a case report and review of the literature. *Int J Gynecol Cancer*. 2006;16:391-3.

199. Takahashi T, Higashi S, Nishiyama H, et al. Biweekly paclitaxel and gemcitabine for patients with advanced urothelial cancer ineligible for cisplatin-based regimen. *Jpn J Clin Oncol*. 2006;36:104-8.

200. Leimgruber K, Negro R, Baier S, et al. Fatal interstitial pneumonitis associated with docetaxel administration in a patient with hormone-refractory prostate cancer. *Tumori*. 2006;92:542-4.

201. Kouroussis C, Mavroudis D, Kakolyris S, et al. High incidence of pulmonary toxicity of weekly docetaxel and gemcitabine in patients with non-small cell lung cancer: results of a dose-finding study. *Lung Cancer*. 2004;44:363-8.

202. Ramanathan R, Reddy VV, Holbert JM, et al. Pulmonary infiltrates following administration of paclitaxel. *Chest*. 1996;110:289-92.

203. Wong P, Leung AN, Berry GJ, et al. Paclitaxel-induced hypersensitivity pneumonitis: radiographic and CT findings. *Am J Roentgenol*. 2001;176:718-20.

204. Rajkumar SV, Hayman S, Gertz MA, et al. Combination therapy with thalidomide plus dexamethasone for newly diagnosed myeloma. *J Clin Oncol*. 2002;20:4319-23.

205. Gordinier ME, Dizon DS. Dyspnea during thalidomide treatment for advanced ovarian cancer. *Ann Pharmacother*. 2005;39:962-5.

206. Curley MJ, Hussein SA, Hassoun PM. Disseminated herpes simplex virus and varicella zoster virus coinfection in a patient taking thalidomide for relapsed multiple myeloma. *J Clin Microbiol*. 2002;40:2302-4.

207. Bennett CL, Schumock GT, Desai AA, et al. Thalidomide-associated deep vein thrombosis and pulmonary embolism. *Am J Med*. 2002;113:603-6.

208. Iguchi T, Sakoda M, Chen CK, et al. Interstitial pneumonia during treatment with thalidomide in a patient with multiple myeloma. *Rinsho Ketsueki*. 2004;45:1064-6.

209. Onozawa M, Hashino S, Sogabe S, et al. Side effects and good effects from new chemotherapeutic agents: Case 2. Thalidomide-induced interstitial pneumonitis. *J Clin Oncol*. 2005;23:2425-6.

Index

Please note page numbers with *f* and *t* indicate figure and table respectively.